# Annotated Psychotherapy

*Annotated Psychotherapy* demonstrates how an experienced psychotherapist develops and carries out the right treatment plan through interactions with the patient or client. In these pages, clinicians will find an explanation of everything the therapist says to patients or clients: why they say it, what they intend it to do, how it fits in with the treatment plan for that person, and, importantly, what might have been said that would be better.

Each of the eight sessions are presented in the form of a transcript that shows how a seasoned clinician might conduct the session—what their internal judgments are and what reasoning or rationale they might have for the therapeutic interventions they choose. Discussion sections after each transcript and a glossary provide helpful explanatory material for the key ideas and concepts, making this book an enlightening resource for therapists working and training in psychotherapy, whether their background is psychology, social work, psychiatry, or counseling.

**Richard B. Makover**, a lecturer at the Yale School of Medicine, developed his psychotherapy concepts in private practice and as clinical director of mental health services at a large health maintenance organization in Connecticut.

"Have you ever wished to observe the work of a therapist first-hand? This comprehensive guide provides a bird's eye view of therapy and the therapeutic assessment process. *Annotated Psychotherapy* is a handy reference and a complete package that offers not only therapy transcripts and therapist evaluative comments but also explanations of key therapy concepts and a glossary of terms. Reading it is almost like having a supervisor by your side as you develop your therapeutic skills."

**Ann Goelitz, PhD, LCSW**, *psychotherapist and author of* From Trauma to Healing: A Social Worker's Guide to Working with Survivors, 2nd edition, *and* Shared Mass Trauma in Social Work: Implications and Strategies for Resilient Practice

"This book, with its unique format of annotated transcripts of therapy sessions, is a valuable addition to the library of resources available to psychotherapists of all disciplines and will be especially useful in training new therapists."

**Robert Rohrbaugh, MD**, *professor of psychiatry and associate dean of global health education at Yale School of Medicine*

"*Annotated Psychotherapy* reveals the therapist's internal dialogue in reaction to patient's statements. The valuable lesson of the book is how the dialogue serves to guide the therapist to adjust the delivery of the psychotherapy. *Annotated Psychotherapy* joins Makover's *Treatment Planning for Psychotherapists* and *Basics of Psychotherapy* to create an essential foundation for educating therapists."

**Diane Sholomskas, PhD**, *assistant clinical professor of psychiatry at the Yale School of Medicine and codirector of the Center for Treatment of Anxiety Disorders and Phobias*

# Annotated Psychotherapy

## A Session by Session Look at How a Therapist Thinks

Richard B. Makover

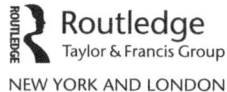

Routledge
Taylor & Francis Group

NEW YORK AND LONDON

Designed cover image: © Yifet Fang / Getty Images

First published 2024
by Routledge
605 Third Avenue, New York, NY 10158

and by Routledge
4 Park Square, Milton Park, Abingdon, Oxon, OX14 4RN

*Routledge is an imprint of the Taylor & Francis Group, an informa business*

*Library of Congress Cataloging-in-Publication Data*
Names: Makover, Richard B., 1938- author.
Title: Annotated psychotherapy : a session by session look at how a therapist thinks / Richard B. Makover.
Description: New York, NY : Routledge, 2024. | Includes bibliographical references and index.
Identifiers: LCCN 2023005230 (print) | LCCN 2023005231 (ebook) | ISBN 9781032398471 (hardback) | ISBN 9781032398440 (paperback) | ISBN 9781003353003 (ebook)
Subjects: LCSH: Psychotherapy—Case studies.
Classification: LCC RC465 .M27 2024 (print) | LCC RC465 (ebook) | DDC 616.89/14—dc23/eng/20230503
LC record available at https://lccn.loc.gov/2023005230
LC ebook record available at https://lccn.loc.gov/2023005231

ISBN: 9781032398471 (hbk)
ISBN: 9781032398440 (pbk)
ISBN: 9781003353003 (ebk)

DOI: 10.4324/9781003353003

Typeset in Times New Roman
by Deanta Global Publishing Services, Chennai, India

Dedication: Henry B. Makover, MD (1908–1987)

The Moving Finger writes; and having writ,
Moves on: nor all thy Piety nor Wit
Shall lure it back to cancel half a Line
Nor all thy Tears wash out a Word of it.

Edward Fitzgerald, *The Rubáiyát of Omar Khayyám*

# Contents

# Permissions

# Author's Disclaimer

# About the Author

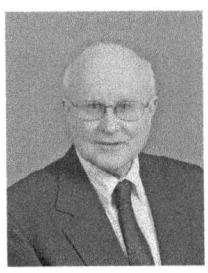 **Richard B. Makover** graduated from Yale University and the Albert Einstein College of Medicine. After a year as a medical intern, he completed his psychiatric training as chief resident, served as a psychiatrist in the United States Navy and then opened a private practice. He was appointed to academic posts at Cornell University Medical College and at New York Medical College. He served as president of a child guidance clinic and chairman of a program review committee for Connecticut's Department of Mental Retardation. His administrative experience includes chairmanship of a hospital psychiatry department, chief of a neuropsychiatry service, and clinical director of psychiatry at a large health maintenance organization. He has been a consultant in geriatric psychiatry and worked extensively in the field of sleep medicine. Drawing on his widespread clinical experience, in 1996 he proposed a new system of treatment planning. That book, *Treatment Planning for Psychotherapists*, is in its revised 3rd edition. In 2017 he published a textbook, *Basics of Psychotherapy*. He is currently a lecturer at the Yale School of Medicine Department of Psychiatry. He lives in Connecticut with his wife, Janet.

# Introduction

A psychotherapist in full-time clinical practice might see six to eight clients a day and carry a caseload of 20 to 30 clients per week.[1] Experienced therapists, although they may be trained in a range of different methodologies, manage this workload by reliance on their basic proficiencies, the group of principles and procedures that apply to generic psychotherapy, the essential competencies that they may employ in a variety of clinical challenges.

This fundamental set of proficiencies is usually concentrated in areas of communication and the analytic examination of patient behaviors, skills that need to be learned during a therapist's years of training. If they are not adequately prepared, however, therapists must hope to hone these skills after their formal education through further study and supervised experience, only to find that those opportunities and the time to devote to them are both in short supply.

Other health care providers are trained, in part, through an apprentice model that allows them many opportunities to observe first-hand how senior experts in their field think about and provide services. A surgeon in training assists at operations. An experienced physical therapist demonstrates procedures to a beginning PT. A student nurse shadows the duties of a registered nurse. Medical students watch residents and attendings perform hands-on treatment. In all these teaching opportunities, the apprentice is:

- Physically present as the care is provided.
- Hears the expert explain the treatment as it takes place.

DOI: 10.4324/9781003353003-1

- Sees first-hand what is being done as it happens.
- Is able to question the expert in real time.

With these advantages, trainees learn from an experienced practitioner not only what to do and how to do it but when and why it is done.

In behavioral health programs, however, the prospects for apprentice learning are limited. Trainees often have few opportunities to discover how experienced therapists think and how they interact with their clients. They may discuss their own patient/client sessions with a supervisor but time pressure restricts their review to a few key points. They may watch a senior therapist (through one-way glass or on a video) but, as silent outside observers, they cannot appreciate the demonstrator's internal judgments and reasoning or examine the specific rationale for each of the therapeutic interventions.

Consider a training demonstration in which a senior therapist interviews a volunteer client while watched by a group of therapists in training. The observers see the two participants sitting across from one another. They hear the client's monologue and the therapist's responses. They witness the non-verbal behaviors of both participants. Unmeasured, but significant nonetheless, is the effect their viewing of the demonstration has on its validity, the observer effect. Do either of the two participants, both aware of the audience, behave as they would alone? Probably not.

The value of these clinical demonstrations often lies in the global effect on the observers. They may choose to model themselves after the style and the technique exhibited in the interview. They may pick up and store away a particular turn of phrase or interview technique. What they miss, however, is the real-time, moment-to-moment knowledge of what the therapist is thinking or why she or he makes those remarks to the client. What is lacking, in other words, is the most important part of the demonstration, the therapist's cognitive process. Even in the discussion after the interview, the therapist instructor will only be able to provide general explanations for his or her responses to the client and not the detailed, relevant ideas that lay behind each one. And despite their instructional value most training programs can provide only a limited number of these demonstrations. Inevitably, as therapists graduate and begin their careers even these minimal eyewitness opportunities vanish.

The demonstrations presented in the annotated sessions to follow attempt to duplicate the apprentice experience. The therapy transcripts include immediate commentary that provides access to the therapist's moment-to-moment assessment and decision processes. To lay the groundwork for these transcripts, the next two chapters examine some of the concepts needed to make full use of the annotations. "General Principles of Psychotherapy" discusses the basic principles and practices that support the diversity of therapeutic systems. It includes a discussion of the importance of formulation in treatment planning. "Therapeutic Communication" reviews some of the therapist's specialized communication skills.

The clinical chapters that follow present one or two sessions with eight patients seen by the therapist, Jane. She has been in private practice for ten years. She spends one day a week at a mental health clinic associated with the local hospital where she supervises trainees and also sees two or three patients for individual psychotherapy. She holds a clinical appointment at the nearby university. Her connection with the school enhances her professional standing and it provides opportunities for contact with other professionals. She has an eclectic approach to her work, utilizing a variety of therapeutic strategies based on what she thinks the patient needs and what she feels comfortable in providing.

To avoid clutter, some of the terminology and technical concepts used in the annotations (identified in small caps) are defined in the Glossary. These terms illustrate the diverse nature of modern therapy: they draw on directive, exploratory and experiential treatment approaches used by therapists who want to be prepared to deal with a wide spectrum of patients and their particular problems.

These case examples comprise only a sample of the many life situations and personal problems that therapists encounter. Taken together, they nevertheless demonstrate many of the common challenges that arise in psychotherapy. Following how Jane thinks about each session will illuminate how a therapist with a treatment plan deals with the moment-to-moment vicissitudes of the therapeutic relationship. Jane is experienced and competent but sometimes she misses a clinical opening or makes a misstep. Readers may learn as much from these occasional oversights as they can when she is successful.

## Note

1   What to call the people who seek our help varies among different practitioners. Some prefer the term "client," because it better reflects the collaborative nature of their work together. Given my medical background, the term "patient" occurs more naturally to me, even though I agree that collaboration is essential to any psychotherapy. I use the two terms interchangeably throughout this book.

# General Principles of Psychotherapy

This chapter discusses the basic principles, the underlying structure of the variety of behavioral health services that fall under the general heading of psychotherapy. The ideas in this chapter and the next apply to what all the many systems of psychotherapy share in common.

## What Is Psychotherapy?

Psychotherapy is the inclusive name for a diverse group of interpersonal services that encompasses a wide-ranging variety of named treatment approaches. One survey, conducted almost three decades ago, documented over 400 different behavioral treatment systems all identifying themselves as psychotherapy (Bergin & Garfield, 1994). Imagine how that list has expanded since! In general, psychotherapy is the service we therapists offer to people who want to improve their future. The past cannot be altered. The present only provides a foundation for modification. We hope our collaborative efforts will help them, going forward, to achieve an enhanced and more successful life.

All those many psychotherapies are united in one common purpose: to offer the prospect of improving problematic behaviors. In some cases, these difficulties have been characterized as a mental disorder (American Psychiatric Association, 2022) or even a mental illness. For many people, however, the problems with which they struggle do not rise to the level of a named disorder, even though the sufferer might have certain character traits or even symptoms that are listed in published compilations of these diagnoses. Recognition of how widespread these

DOI: 10.4324/9781003353003-2

problems can be has led to the retitling of mental health services as behavioral health services. This revision makes sense because the fundamental purpose of psychotherapy is not to improve *mental* functioning—a slippery concept that is hard to define— but instead to achieve more effective and rewarding behaviors. While other phenomena may shift during therapy—perceptions, feelings, insight, emotional stability, even self-image—they are relevant only if they facilitate the behavior change that defines the desired outcome.

The main difference among these many disciplines, in addition to their theoretical foundations, is where they fall along a continuum of methodological structure. For example, dialectical behavior therapy (DBT) is highly structured and multifaceted (Dimeff & Linehan, 2001), while psychoanalytic psychotherapy is relatively unstructured and widely focused (Marcus, 2002). Each of this multitude of therapies will usually fit into one of three general categories:

*Directive therapies* follow a protocol that asks the client to undertake particular tasks or to follow certain procedures designed to address target symptoms. Cognitive-behavioral therapy (CBT) is an example of the directive type (Craske, 2017).

*Exploratory therapies* look for the precursors and underlying sources of current behavior with the hope that exposing them to the patient's examination will effect improvements in problematic areas. An example of the exploratory type is psychodynamic psychotherapy (Cabaniss, 2016).

*Experiential therapies* use expressive techniques to help clients recreate, connect with and alter harmful influences from the past, using role-playing, artistic activities, music and the like to bring those influences under present control. Gestalt therapy is an example (Wheeler & Axelsson, 2017).

In practice, however, these three categories often overlap. A therapy that begins with a directive protocol may soon need an exploratory technique to deal with issues outside of the original symptoms.

A psychodynamic approach might require a role-playing exercise to overcome a specific problem. An experiential approach based on current behavior could require a cognitive-behavioral protocol to make further progress.

No one can be proficient in all 400-plus psychotherapies. Familiarity and ease with several, however, is usually worthwhile. Jane, the therapist featured in subsequent chapters, knows and uses around half a dozen. Her *eclectic* approach to psychotherapy, utilizing a variety of strategies, allows Jane to help more patients.

## Common Features of All Psychotherapies

Despite their many differences and wide variety of principles and practices, all types of psychotherapy share certain essential qualities. The three most important of these elements are the *placebo effect*, the *nonspecific healing forces* and the presence of *therapeutic change agents*. These common elements may be necessary for the success of the treatment but no one alone is sufficient to ensure a favorable outcome.

### The Placebo Effect

Sometimes called the placebo response, this feature refers to the beneficial effect obtained from an inert or inactive treatment.[1] In general medicine, this remedy is sometimes called a "sugar pill." Although the placebo itself has no scientific therapeutic rationale, it often effects real change. For example, a sugar pill given as an analgesic can alleviate arthritis pain for long periods (Zhang, 2019). Even surgical interventions can turn out to succeed because of the placebo effect. This surprising result was discovered when surgeons treating angina (cardiac-induced chest pain) found the same benefit resulted from a sham (placebo) surgery as from the actual internal mammary artery ligation that had been a standard treatment for this symptom (Miller, 2012).

Legitimate trials of new drugs and treatments always include an inert alternative against which to measure the medication's benefits. The results of clinical drug trials frequently show that the placebo alone accomplished a surprising portion, sometimes as much as 40% or more, of the expected benefit. The tested drug or treatment must show it is significantly better than the placebo before it is approved for general use.

In psychotherapy, the placebo effect often shows up early in treatment as the patient's presenting symptoms improve before any real therapeutic work has been accomplished. In fact, patients on a waiting list may already begin to feel better, apparently in anticipation of treatment that has yet to begin (Endicott & Endicott, 1963). Throughout therapy, this factor may accelerate progress because of the patient's expectation of benefit.[2]

The placebo effect may work by mobilizing the intrinsic tendency toward self-healing that characterizes all living beings. In psychotherapy, it seems to originate from the hopeful possibilities stimulated by the prospect of professional help from an expert practitioner. Any elements of the psychotherapy experience are likely to enhance these effects and may lead to permanent benefits.

- The initial interview may provide such hopeful expectations because the therapist comes across as professional, competent, knowledgeable and concerned.
- Early progress, such as the elimination of unrealistic worries or an appreciation of the therapist's understanding of the identified troubles may result in the disappearance of or at least a reduction in some presenting problems.
- Even personal characteristics, as perceived by the new client, may have a placebo effect. The good reputation of the therapist, the professional surroundings of the office environment and the professional appearance of the therapist, the perceived confidence that the therapist can help, or the association of the therapist with a respected institution—all may contribute to early progress.

While the placebo effect may be more significant at the beginning of therapy, its continuing influence plus the new developments that continue to stimulate it can persist through the entire treatment period.

The placebo effect is sometimes regarded as a counterfeit benefit, one that is not based on actual change, but this notion ignores the way emotional expectancies can modify the way experiences are integrated into general behavior. Hopeful expectation can lead to real and permanent change. Optimism fuels progress.

### Nonspecific Factors

We can broaden the idea of "psychotherapy" to encompass a variety of healing activities that promote the recovery from psychological impairment. These might include:

- Unconventional approaches such as faith healing, religious revivalism and the immersion in cults.
- Various magic ceremonies that incorporate the supernatural and its rites, such as calling upon spirits or casting spells.
- The mundane material provided in self-help books, some of which recycle simple ideas and obvious solutions but which nevertheless continually find a willing audience. For example, *How to Stop Worrying and Start Living* by Dale Carnegie, published 75 years ago, is still in print and selling today (Carnegie, 1948).
- And, of course, all the different systems of psychotherapy.

The common elements linking these seemingly disparate areas comprise a nonspecific set of forces first noted by Jerome Frank.

In *Persuasion and Healing*, Frank identified four shared characteristics that were common to all of these different modalities (Frank & Frank, 1991):

- The first characteristic was a *relationship* with another person who was perceived to have the ability to bring healing forces to bear. The bond with the healer must be one that encourages open, revealing speech and the expression of emotion. The healer might as easily be an evangelical preacher, a tribal shaman or a self-help author as a widely published psychotherapist.[3]

- The healing activity had to occur in a special safe *environment* that validated the healer's prestige and competence. The setting could be an isolated commune or an outdoor revival meeting under a tent or a magic circle made from a ring of stones or an office in a professional building: all of them convey the safety of a protected sanctuary.
- The activity must occur in the context of an explanation that made sense of the sufferer's ordeal. Frank called the explanation the *myth*, perhaps to include the wide variety of logical and irrational features each typically contains.[4] The "myth" could be the potency of a sacred amulet or the soul-saving act of confession or the power of unconscious mental forces.
- Finally, all of the varied efforts had to include a procedure, an articulated system, that could be employed to guide the sufferer through the recovery into health. Frank called this feature the *ritual*. Equivalent processes might be a ceremonial baptism or handling venomous snakes while speaking in tongues or the acceptance of the psychoanalytic couch.

Relationship, environment, myth and ritual do not evoke the practical realities of 21st century life. The comparisons between psychotherapy and such religious, magical or self-help practices that lack an accepted scientific basis may strike the modern reader as inappropriate if not distasteful. It might help to keep in mind that the human brain has undergone little change over the last 200,000 years, a mere flicker of evolutionary time. We possess the same drive to pursue patterns and meanings and experience the same swarm of emotions as did the earliest Homo sapiens. No surprise then that we have the same responses to myth and ritual as our progenitors. Perhaps the parallels are less disconcerting if we acknowledge that emotional forces and the effect of various traumas on our psyches are as potent now as they were when humans were hunter-gatherers living in tribes whose daily existence was always under threat. Today, we can be grateful that, with a willing, patient and a skillful therapist, these ancient dynamics can be mobilized to help improve the lives of modern sufferers.

In any case, the parallels between Frank's identified nonspecific factors and modern psychotherapy are clear:

- We take on the mantle of healer when we present ourselves as competent, recognized therapists. Our social standing is bolstered by the assumption that we have the special training of our profession and is further supported by the certification of a professional accreditation and by a license issued through a controlling government agency. These external attributes justify and sanction the *relationship* we offer to our patients and clients.
- Our activities typically take place in a closed, pleasant space, usually our office, that can be soundproofed and protected from intrusion for the duration of the meeting with our sufferer. We provide privacy and, within certain legal limits, confidentiality. Thus, we fulfill the requirements for a special safe *environment*.[5]
- We typically provide a description or a diagnosis of sorts for the identified psychological issues we propose to treat. While our particular account may differ from what might be offered by a therapist with a different theoretical stance, our explanation will be internally consistent and, hopefully, persuasive. In other words, our sufferer is invited to accept our *myth*.
- The sufferer learns, either through our direct educational efforts or from experiencing the conduct of the therapy, that we have a set of procedures, a coherent methodology, that will be followed to achieve the desired healing. The range of procedures in psychotherapy is wide, encompassing free association, meeting with a group of fellow sufferers, painting one's feelings on canvas or role-playing a past trauma. This process constitutes our *ritual*.

So, rather than begrudge the comparison between our own professional activities and the somewhat fringe or suspect status of the other varieties of persuasive healing, perhaps we should be more confident in our own approaches, knowing that they occur against a background of historical success over millennia of interpersonal healing.

### Therapeutic Change Agents

The last of the common elements found in all psychotherapies were clearly identified by T. Byram Karasu and comprise three necessary healing forces (Karasu, 1986):

- The first nonspecific healing force Karasu called *affective experiencing*. Behavioral problems contain emotional content. For example, a simple phobia, say, fear of spiders, means that the expectation of meeting a spider or seeing one in proximity to oneself elicits anxiety, dread, disgust. These strong feelings must be disarmed in the course of treating the phobia.

  The more subtle or widespread problems that might bring someone to a therapist come with their own set of affects and require the same attention and eventual resolution for the treatment to succeed. These emotions may emerge as a sudden strong release (catharsis or abreaction) or they may simmer along within the regular therapy work. Attention to the affective experiences of the patient is needed to remove barriers to change and to enhance new, more adaptive behaviors.

- *Cognitive mastery* is the second prerequisite for treatment success. Here Karasu recognizes the same requirement as in Frank's theoretical system or *the myth*. In both classifications, the methodology provides an intellectual framework that creates a rational understanding for the origin and impact of the target behaviors. A psychodynamic approach may identify early childhood traumas that manifest as current difficulties. A cognitive-behavioral analysis might focus on antecedent forces that lead to cognitive distortion. An existential therapy may emphasize the need to accept the realities of human survival. In all cases, the rational basis provided by the therapy system is used to guide the treatment toward a favorable result. The ability of the sufferer to understand the problematic behavior, not as a mysterious, uncontrollable set of forces, but rather as an identifiable, rational, explainable set of circumstances provides the sense of control (of "mastery") that promotes the desired recovery and healing.

- Karasu identified the third requirement as *behavioral regulation*. Here he recognized that actual, persistent positive change in behavior is the unique measure of treatment success. As mentioned in the definition given earlier, effective psychotherapy, regardless of its many systems and methods, requires a helpful and stable change from maladaptive to successful behaviors.

    More specifically, this principle of behavioral regulation rejects the significance of the common, highly valued features of a particular psychotherapy system. Examples might include insight produced by a psychodynamic therapy or the recognition of overgeneralized thoughts in a CBT protocol or the acceptance of the inevitability that life ends developed within an existential therapy. These are real achievements, but they are only provisional steps toward the hoped-for emergence of stable new behaviors that constitute the treatment goals.

    In too many cases, however, the patient remains in treatment for long periods, steeped in the experience of a particular therapy method, perhaps achieving many of these provisional steps, but absent real behavioral change—with little to no improvement in the problematic behaviors that brought them to the therapist. Lacking the required "behavioral regulation" the therapy fails to achieve its desired aim.

The presence of all three healing forces provides the best opportunity for the desired outcome. If one or more is missing, success becomes more elusive. For example, consider a highly emotional client who never achieves cognitive mastery. Think of an intellectually sophisticated patient who understands the structure and meaning of his problem but fails to generate the appropriate emotional response. Neither is likely to achieve the behavioral changes that would alleviate their troubles.

## The Psychotherapy Relationship

The preceding discussion of the elements of psychotherapy all manifest themselves through the *relationship* between the therapist and the person, family or group who require the therapist's services. In fact, two types are present throughout the therapy: the real relationship and the therapeutic alliance.

### The Real Relationship

The real relationship arises from the administrative and structural demands behind the work of the therapy itself: the non-therapeutic transactions between the two parties. It includes the agreement on a schedule of sessions or even how many sessions will be allowed. It can involve the financial arrangements, including whether they require third-party payments or self-funding, as well as the expectations of when the bills will be due and payable.[6]

Beyond these practical decisions, the real relationship incorporates certain concrete, non-therapeutic expectations. Examples are the recognition that the therapist is paid for services rendered, that therapists have other clients, that they go home at the end of the day, enjoying a separate life outside of the office. Other expectations include: all appointments will be kept. The session will start and end on time. Bills will be paid in a timely fashion. The office environment will be respected.

From time to time, certain aspects of the real relationship will contaminate the therapeutic effort. For example: The client may fail to keep an appointment. The patient may arrive chronically late. The client may not pay the bill. The breakdown in these administrative matters usually means the therapeutic alliance has weakened. It can also indicate that the therapy has failed to address some important aspect of the treatment plan and effort must be diverted from other therapy efforts to address and correct the omission.

### The Therapeutic Alliance

The professional relationship between the participants in psychotherapy is termed the therapeutic alliance.[7] It refers to the commitment between them that together they will overcome the behavioral difficulties that are the agreed focus of the treatment. Disruption of the therapeutic alliance often results in treatment failure and in clients leaving therapy prematurely (Homan, 2019).

The therapeutic alliance is the result of contributions from both the therapist and the client. The therapist brings such personal assets as warmth, sincerity, flexibility, tolerance, openness, empathy, integrity and concern for the client. The client provides, among other things, emotional intelligence, motivation, trust and a willingness to cooperate. The safe environment, such as the office, contributes to the confidence between them that the work can succeed.

This alliance alone will usually account for some of the progress the patient makes regardless of the psychotherapy procedure itself. How much it contributes is a matter of speculation and percentages vary. My own estimate is that it accounts for around 50% of the success of the therapy. Assuming that to be true, it suggests that even the most poorly run course of treatment—poorly run from a technical perspective, that is—will still accomplish half the job, *provided the therapeutic alliance is strong*. The other 50% depends on the accuracy of the formulation, the precision of the treatment plan and the skill of the therapist. While it may be a comfort that half the job is already assured by the therapeutic alliance, professional satisfaction can only result from the sense that everything possible has been accomplished.

## Beginning Treatment

Every course of treatment begins when the therapist first encounters the person who is seeking help. This encounter should comprehend four steps that will help ensure a successful outcome:[8]

- First, an *initial evaluation* that allows the therapist to assess the prospect's motivation and suitability for treatment and to identify the problems on which the therapy should focus.
- Second, a *formulation* or analysis of those problems within whatever intellectual framework the therapist relies on for understanding.

- Third, the construction of a *treatment plan* that encompasses the therapy's goals and hoped-for outcomes.
- Fourth, an *agreement* with the client on how they will accomplish its goals.

This section briefly examines each of the four steps.

### The Initial Evaluation

In this short summary, it is difficult to cover the many tasks and complex decision-making included in the initial interview. The reader may want to consult the many other sources of information on this topic.[9]

The first meeting between the two participants is often a semi-structured interview that permits the patient to lay out the background of the presenting problems while it also allows the therapist to gain the required facts of the case through direct questions. Additional information might include the referral materials and the records of prior treatment.

An important datum is to determine what it is that the client *wants* from therapy. This question is usually neither simple nor obvious, and what is wanted may not be the therapeutic benefit the therapist hopes to offer. One study (Frank et al., 1978) compiled a list of over a dozen different requests, including such things as:

- Clarification. A client, referred by someone else, may seek a better understanding of their supposed problem, perhaps hoping to be told there is none.
- Ventilation. The patient may want a sympathetic auditor, possibly someone who will agree the fault lies with others.
- Control. The client could perceive the therapy relationship as a power struggle and be determined to win it.
- Confession. The patient may hope for relief merely by revealing things in confidence that cannot be said elsewhere, with no motivation for behavioral change.
- Nothing. The client was coerced into treatment by someone else, a spouse or even a court, and has no intention of cooperating.[10]

It may take considerable effort to elicit a covert agenda but the additional work is a critical element of the initial assessment. For therapy to reach a successful outcome therapist and client must agree that what the client wants is something the therapist can and will provide.

The initial interview should culminate in a coherent history leading to an initial understanding of what the patient needs. It should include a mental status evaluation, especially with an assessment of risk as to suicidal or other potentially harmful behavior, although many of the mental status data points can be assessed without formal questions. The sum of all the information-gathering should result in a clear idea of what needs to be accomplished.

### *Formulation*

An important but often overlooked feature of the initial interview is the formulation. Using the information gathered, and with a background of psychological knowledge, the therapist can identify what caused the problems that the therapy is expected to resolve. The intellectual framework for this understanding can be any of the psychological models that underlie the different therapeutic modalities. In other words, it could be psychodynamics, or cognitive-behavioral theory or any of the humanistic systems. So long as the result is a coherent explanation, based on cause and effect, the formulation will be useful in deciding how to proceed with treatment.

In medical practice, a standard part of the evaluation is a *differential diagnosis*, a rank ordering of all the diagnostic possibilities suggested by the patient's signs and symptoms. This listing leads to a series of tests and other procedures that will rule in or rule out diagnostic possibilities until, hopefully, only one—the most likely of the lot—becomes the correct diagnosis. The validity of these tests relies on the scientific understanding of the underlying pathology that presents as a medical disease.

Tests and procedures for psychological assessment are far less useful. They comprise a variety of instruments, often in the form of questionnaires, to help screen, diagnose and monitor various conditions. In an evaluation for psychotherapy, however, these written instruments may not be practical or dispositive. Like the taxonomy of diagnostic categories, they rely on descriptions of patient symptoms. Lacking the body of scientific data that underlies medical testing, however, they can only confirm a descriptive category or bolster the therapist's judgment about symptom severity. When administered, they take time away from the face-to-face interaction so important to establishing a therapeutic alliance. Perhaps their main value is to provide research data or a concrete basis for insurance claims or for medicolegal purposes. In real-world terms, the practicing therapist will usually rely on making a best judgment based on the history and mental status alone.

Formulation is a challenge because it requires inductive reasoning. Unlike the more familiar deductive process, *the more information presented the harder the inductive task*. In deductive reasoning, the kind needed to arrive at a diagnosis, for instance, the more facts available the easier it is to reach a conclusion. A diagnosis is based on identification of the individual elements that define it. If the only symptom is "anorexia," for example, the number of possible diagnostic categories is large (dieting, bulimia, chemotherapy, depression, delusional disorder and more), but add hopelessness, early morning awakening, anhedonia and suicidal ideation and the diagnosis of major depression begins to emerge.

Inductive reasoning, however, requires building a single abstract concept out of a collection of data. The more items available the harder it is to find the specific group into which they all fit. For example, consider the pair: a banana and an orange. The obvious category is "fruit." Now add oatmeal and coffee. The four items may be grouped as "breakfast food" but they might also be "things I need from the supermarket" or even "foods I don't like to eat." The answer, at least, is less obvious than for only the two items. Add further: Grandma's cookie recipe and a crock pot. Perhaps the category for all six items is now "things found in the kitchen," certainly a more vague and tentative conclusion than before. An initial interview may reveal a list of 10 or 20 disparate items of history and current symptoms, making the effort to contain them in a single useful set a challenging task.

A shortcut to this process is a list of categories that covers most of the psychotherapy topics into which the available facts may be incorporated. In effect, this exercise turns the difficult process of induction into the easier mode of deduction. Here are some categories with descriptions:

| | |
|---|---|
| Biological | Disorders with a known or likely organic basis. |
| Developmental | Troubled transition between phases of adult maturation. |
| Dissociative | Complications from abuse, neglect or other trauma. |
| Situational | Stress-related symptoms with inadequate coping skills. |
| Transactional | Social difficulties arising from interpersonal dysfunction. |
| Existential | Responses to isolation and death. |
| Psychodynamic | Irrational behavior reflecting intrapsychic problems. |

Using these seven likely areas of difficulty, most patient histories can be categorized in a way that leads to an inductive conclusion about what needs to be done in the recommended therapy.

### Treatment Plans

Using the history and the formulation, therapists should be able to identify the areas of behavioral dysfunction that will be the focus of treatment. These ideas can then be developed into a concrete plan of treatment.

The plan begins with a decision about what should be the overall desired outcome (the AIM) of the treatment. As noted above and as the examples suggest, the therapist may determine that what the client *wants* is something inappropriate or unattainable. For example, a client, considering divorce, may want the therapist's agreement that the spouse is responsible for a bad marriage, while the therapist may have recognized distortions in the client's perceptions and the ways the client has created unnecessary problems in the relationship. These observations could form the basis of a workable treatment plan. They must then discuss and negotiate until what the client wants and what the therapist is willing to accept are congruent, if not exactly the same.[11]

Next, the therapist must decide what has to be accomplished (the GOALS) in order to reach this outcome and which of the available therapeutic approaches (the STRATEGIES) might best reach them. The final step is to select the specific techniques (the TACTICS) needed to carry out a strategy.[12]

In outline form, a treatment plan might look like that in Figure 2.1.

In this example three distinct goals are required to reach a successful outcome. Each goal needs its strategy and tactics, although goals 2 and 3 both need strategy 3.

Suppose, for example, that the *aim* for a depressed patient with a poor employment history was to help overcome the mood disorder.

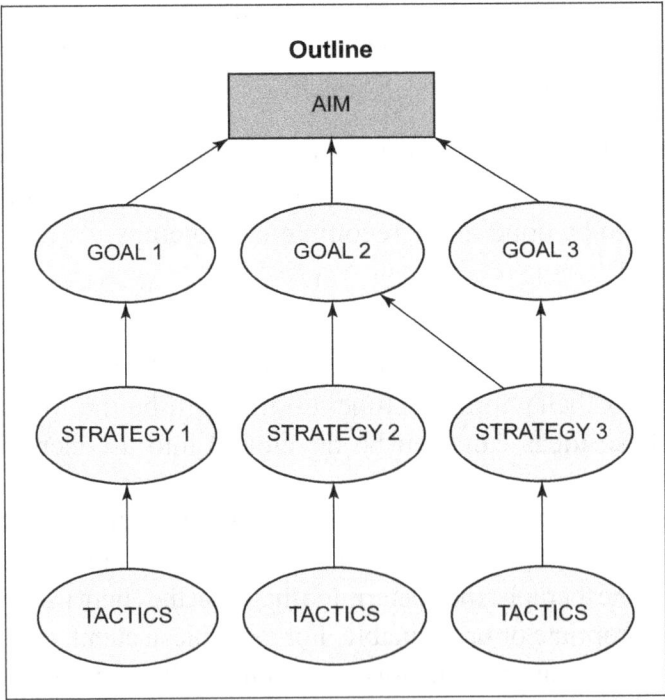

*Figure 2.1* Complex treatment planning diagram Source: From *Treatment Planning for Psychotherapists*, 3rd edition, by Richard B. Makover, © 2016. Used by permission of American Psychiatric Association Publishing.

It might require a course of antidepressant medication to reach *goal 1* (a normalized mood), a clinical case management (directive) approach to deal with the employment problem (*goal 2*), and a cognitive-behavioral examination of the depressive ruminations that accompany the illness (*goal 3*). CBT is a *strategy* needed for the ruminations but also for the employment issues. When and how to use these three *strategies* would depend on the flow of each session. Finally, the effective use of any *strategy* requires knowledge of and familiarity with the particular tools of each. For CBT, for example, the *tactic* of exposure and response prevention might be needed.

### The Treatment Contract

The final step in treatment planning is the presentation of the plan to the patient in order to reach an agreement on how therapy will proceed: the *treatment contract*. The contract is usually verbal. Some negotiation may be needed if the patient has different ideas about what should happen. What the patient wants and what the therapist can offer must, in the end, be congruent. The validity and usefulness of the contract depend on the patient's sincerity, openness and honesty. A patient with strong sociopathic traits, for instance, may lack these qualities and the result will be a false contract that will ultimately fail.

It is tempting to skip this step and just move ahead with the planned therapy, but failure to agree on a treatment contract will often result in a poor outcome. If the therapist assumes that an agreement has been reached without overtly confirming what it comprises, the disconnect will often lead to a breakdown of the progress of therapy that becomes a structural impasse. Unless resolved, treatment—at least, effective treatment—will end.

### Modification of Plans

Treatment plans for behavioral health therapies cannot rely on a formal diagnosis. As noted before, the official list of disorders (American Psychiatric Association, 2022) is essentially a collection of descriptions, a taxonomy based on observed characteristics lumped together under separate headings. Human beings are full of contradictions and variations, however, and patients often present with an assortment of symptoms that do not fully match any single diagnostic category or that span several different categories. Instead, accurate assessment of what problems need treatment is better addressed through the formulation, the detailed assessment of what troubles that singular client.

Although the formulation is unique to a particular client, it rests on a more general understanding of human behavior and especially on the deviations from successful behaviors that qualify as symptoms. The specificity of the formulation leads to a treatment plan that recognizes what is the client's maladaptive behavior and that proposes to correct it.

One aspect of human behavior, however, that undermines the integrity of the formulation is that human beings, to be blunt, tend to lie. Mostly, they are lies of omission, as the interviewee leaves out important facts from the history, but lies of commission are also a problem. Lying is organic to the human species: people lie to protect themselves or to maintain or gain social status. They lie in business transactions as well as in intimate relationships. So it should be no surprise that they lie to their therapists. Incorrect and missing data introduces flaws into the formulation that will sometimes seriously encumber treatment plans.

The original formulation relies on the initial history. When additional history or corrections emerge over the course of treatment, the formulation must also evolve and the treatment plan that rests upon it must be modified to reflect that evolution. One hopes that the subsequent formulations represent *successive approximations of the truth* and that therapy becomes more accurate and effective as a result.

## Summary

Psychotherapy, like most of health care, requires not only a scientific knowledge base but also the flexibility and creativity of an experienced practitioner. As with many healing efforts it can be more an art than a science. The therapist who is aware of, and practices within, the historical framework from which it developed may be more successful at helping troubled people find better solutions to their problems.

## Notes

1  The placebo effect can also be harmful, especially when it is appears to support commercial activities that seek to take advantage of the public's naivety. Countless patent medicines and worthless remedies are advertised and sold based on the expectation that the placebo effect will promote some claimed benefit for which there is no scientific basis. People are asked to believe that product X will restore lost memory function, promote lasting weight loss, control pain or overcome sexual dysfunction, to name a few examples. Thanks to the placebo effect some of those claimed benefits can actually occur, but often only temporarily and usually far less than is needed.

2  The recent proliferation of online psychotherapy services, lacking some of the requirements of in-person treatment, may owe their initial success to the placebo effect.

3  An open question is whether computers can fully replace human therapists. At present, they can help implement certain rigid protocols under human supervision. Whether they can ever develop the empathy, flexibility and creativity of a human therapist seems doubtful.

4  He also used the term "demoralization" to characterize the emotional distress and confusion that accompanied the suffering.

5  Remote delivery of psychotherapy ("Tele-Mental Health") surged during the 2020 viral epidemic and may persist because of convenience and increased access. Will those seeking help from a remote location, such as their home, experience it as a safe environment? Will their data be secure? If not, will their therapy be less successful?

6  The real relationship in fee-for-service arrangements also includes the unfortunate temptation to keep clients in treatment beyond the time legitimately required, either because therapy goals have been met or because progress has slowed or stopped or because of a comfortable relationship between the parties that becomes mislabeled as "support." The only remedy to this distortion of ethical principle depends on the practitioner's moral compass.

7  Other terms in use are the working alliance and the psychotherapy relationship.

8  Any experienced supervisor will have noted how often a therapist has missed one or more of these necessary steps when they confront the breakdown or failure of the therapy.

9  For example, Makover (2017).

10  The list of "wants" also included: administrative help; advice; psychodynamic insight; psychological expertise; reality contact; non-psychiatric medical treatment; succor.

11  The agreement also constitutes "informed consent," an important medicolegal element of any treatment.

12  See also Makover (2016).

# References

American Psychiatric Association. (2022). *Diagnostic and Statistical Manual of Mental Disorders, Fifth Edition, Text Revision (DSM-5-TR)*. American Psychiatric Publishing.

Bergin, A. E., & Garfield, S. L. (Eds.). (1994). *Handbook of psychotherapy and behavior change*. Wiley.

Cabaniss, D. L., et al. (2016). *Psychodynamic psychotherapy: A clinical manual* (2nd ed.). Wiley.

Carnegie, D. (1948). *How to stop worrying and start living*. The Chaucer Press.

Craske, M. G. (2017). *Cognitive-behavioral therapy* (Revised Ed.). American Psychological Association.

Dimeff, L., & Linehan, M. M. (2001). Dialectical behavior therapy in a nutshell. *The California Psychologist*, 34, 10–13.

Endicott, N. A., & Endicott, J. (1963). "Improvement" in untreated psychiatric patients. *Archives of General Psychiatry*, 9, 575–585.

Frank, A. W., Eisenthal, S., & Lazare, A. (1978). Are there social class differences in patients' treatment conceptions? *Archives of General Psychiatry*, 35(1), 611–619.

Frank, J. D., & Frank, J. B. (1991). *Persuasion and healing: A comparative study of psychotherapy* (3rd ed.). Johns Hopkins University Press.

Homan, J. B. (2019). *Attrition and psychotherapy*. Portland State University Dissertations and Theses.

Karasu, T. B. (1986). The specificity versus nonspecificity dilemma: Toward identifying therapeutic change agents. *American Journal of Psychiatry*, 143, 687–695.

Makover, R. B. (2016). *Treatment planning for psychotherapists: A practical guide to better outcomes* (3rd ed.). American Psychiatric Association Publishing.

Makover, R. B. (2017). *Basics of psychotherapy: A practical guide to improving clinical success*. American Psychiatric Association Publishing.

Marcus, E. R. (2002). Psychoanalytic psychotherapy. In Herren, M., & Sledge, W. (Eds.), *Encyclopedia of psychotherapy* (pp. 275–296). Academic Press.

Miller, F. G. (2012). The enduring legacy of sham-controlled trials of internal mammary artery ligation. *Progress in Cardiovascular Diseases*, 55(3), 246–250.

Wheeler, G., & Axelsson, L. (2017). *Gestalt therapy* (2nd ed.). American Psychological Association.

Zhang, W. (2019). The powerful placebo effect in osteoarthritis. *Clinical and Experimental Rheumatology*, 37(Suppl. 120), 118–123.

# Therapeutic Communication

Communication between therapist and patient is at the heart of every therapeutic methodology. It is the means to support the therapeutic alliance, to identify and illuminate areas and topics of significance, to mobilize emotion, to overcome resistance, to facilitate behavioral change. The various types of communication are, in effect, the therapist's tools of the trade.

When they employ these tools, therapists themselves become therapeutic instruments. Just as it is not the scalpel that treats a physical problem, it is the surgeon who wields it, so in psychotherapy it is not the theory that helps the patient heal—not the strategies and tactics that make up the treatment process—it is the therapist who chooses how and when to "wield" these tools: which ones to use, the timing of each intervention, and the evaluation of which interventions are effective and which are counterproductive. Just as the surgeon develops the skills to use the scalpel, so must the therapist learn to use the psychotherapy tools available. Among the therapist's tools are words, phrases, questions, statements; in other words, cognitive decisions made in response to the patient's verbal and non-verbal production, within the historical context of that person's unique history.

Ideally, every communication from the therapist should have a therapeutic purpose. To accomplish this difficult goal, the therapist must utilize the cognitive function sometimes called the "observing ego" to monitor the progress of a session and make immediate judgments about what to communicate in response to what the patient says and does. The observing ego, or self-observation,

DOI: 10.4324/9781003353003-3

allows the therapist to assess his or her own responses to the other person and to modify or shape the appropriate response.

Spoken words are only part of the communication process and not always the major factor. The rate of speech, its emotional tone, the posture, facial expression and body movements of the speaker give color and nuance to what is being said. Microexpressions, fleeting changes that may not be consciously recognized by the observer, may reveal emotions that challenge or modulate the literal meaning of the spoken ideas. The non-verbal portion of the message may have unintended consequences in its effect on the listener. The context, the general topic being discussed, can modify its significance. This phenomenon is more fully discussed below under metacommunication.

Communication is a broad and complex subject. This chapter can only briefly review a few of these "tools of the trade." They can be best understood as increasing levels of communicative complexity.

## Diction

Which particular word to use is the therapist's first level of complexity. A client's vocabulary varies with age, intelligence and education. How well that person understands the therapist often rests on the shared meaning of the words chosen to communicate a concept or idea. Use of too simple a word may fail to convey the whole import of the therapist's communication. It might even suggest contempt or disdain. Too complex a word may not be understood. It might even convey intellectual arrogance. The decision about the diction required can usually be judged by listening to the client's vocabulary and adopting the same level of complexity.

In addition to matching the client's diction the therapist must be aware of a word's emotional weight. Each word carries its own affective tone. Consider, for example, the English words mater, mother, mom, mummy and momma. Identical in meaning, they differ in their associations—social, class and ethnic—and thus carry distinctly different emotional overtones.

Word choice is often useful in strengthening the therapeutic alliance. By speaking to the client at his or her own level of education and estimated intelligence[1] the therapist can not only get across ideas more successfully, but can also, as a discussion between intellectual equals, support the client's sense of affinity with the therapist. Communication on the client's level facilitates comprehension and helps to keep the relationship strong.

For example, to express the concept of shading the truth:

- For a client with an advanced degree, you might use the word "mendacious."
- For a college graduate, "deceptive."
- For a high school graduate, "false."
- For an eighth grade dropout, "lying."

The same standard would apply to the choice of examples or reference to cultural ideas.

## Naming, Renaming and Reframing

In the Book of Genesis, Adam has only one job: naming everything God has created.[2] *Naming* remains one of the human mind's essential cognitive operations. This fundamental process plays an important role in psychotherapy. Conferring a name is the therapist's second level of complexity.

To identify an emotion, a life crisis, a relationship, or any other problem that—to the patient—is mysterious, confusing, or unacceptable by giving it a particular name can help the patient deal with it more successfully. For example, a frightening experience of dry mouth, pounding heart and tremors when named "a panic attack" (rather than, say, a heart attack) defines it as a manageable problem with short-term fixes (like rebreathing in a paper bag) and long-term solutions (such as exposure and response prevention).

*Renaming* something is another way to use this communicative tool. It may mean identifying something the client considers a defect to suggest it could instead be a strength. For example, a client who says a timid style of decision-making is a source of missed opportunities might be told that this approach shows an admirable caution or prudence. Renaming is also useful to highlight a problem the client denies or fails to recognize. Using the same example: a client who considers procrastination and wavering uncertainty to be evidence of caution and careful consideration of alternatives might be told that these traits instead suggest unneeded timidity and fear of commitment.

Sometimes a whole experience can be redefined or *reframed* in a way that emphasizes its positive nature, such as characterizing a failure that has sapped the patient's confidence and sparked a social withdrawal as, instead, a useful learning experience. Doing so may allow the patient to explore the reasons for the failure unimpeded by guilt and self-hatred.

These three interventions, utilizing the Biblical act of naming, represent the therapist's ability to shape perceptions and self-images that underlie some maladaptive behavioral problems. This influence must be employed with caution and humility, since, used unwisely, it can cause as much harm as good.

## Asking Questions

The form of intervention used is the third level of complexity: whether to intervene by a declaration or an interrogatory. In other words, should the therapist clearly state whatever conclusion has been reached or is it better to tentatively advance the idea in the form of a question? While both forms have their uses, in many cases asking a question is more likely to engage the client than will stating a conclusion.

A direct statement puts the therapist in an authoritarian stance, speaking as an expert, already knowing the answer. A question recognizes a tentative idea that requires confirmation, an open-ended inquiry between collaborating partners in the search for facts. It invites the client's participation in the quest for helpful truths and is more likely to lead to agreement.

For example: "Do you think you were angry when you said that?" or, "You must have been angry when you said that." The first version, asking a question, acknowledges that the client might know what feeling prompted the belligerent statement better than the therapist and invites further explanation. The second version, a flat statement, presumes the therapist knows why it was said, leaving the client with a choice to agree or disagree. Collaboration is less likely and, worst case, the assertion might easily be taken as a criticism, provoking further conflict.

This choice applies across all the different forms psychotherapy might take. In every case, sooner or later, the therapist reaches a conclusion about the patient's behavior, especially one touching on one of the therapy goals, and wants to bring it to the patient's attention. Even when following a prescriptive protocol, such as might be used in a CBT program, it will often be more effective to present the idea in the form of a question, rather than to make a declarative statement.

Human nature tends to resist authority; we don't like to be pushed around, even by a new idea. The possible exception, those who masochistically want to be dominated, nevertheless may find some passive-aggressive way to avoid full compliance. A confident conclusion can provoke some clients to feel pressured or bullied. Others may falsely agree due to passive compliance or misplaced deference. Declarative statements tend to excite the client's resistance, often leading to denial or diversion from the topic or inciting disagreement.

To ask a question also admits the possibility that the allegation may be wrong. The therapist might have a high degree of confidence in the assertion and yet still be incorrect. The data on which it is based could be flawed because clients prevaricate, either by omission or commission. Memory is often incomplete or modified by later experience. The emotions associated with the data may distort its accuracy. More information may emerge in future sessions that will alter the prior conclusion. Given all these possible sources of error it only makes sense to advance one's ideas as tentative possibilities. Therapists should view their explanations with humility.

## "Why" Questions

An exception to the use of questions, however, are some beginning with the word "why." Why questions often have negative implications, whether intended or not (Karasu, 2013), especially those questions that ask about motive. For example, if you, a male therapist, ask a man, "why did you wear that tie today?" he may assume you disapprove of the choice and have no sense of proper style, even if you merely wanted to know if you should have worn a tie yourself. Why questions tend to undermine the therapeutic alliance.

Since it might still be preferable to ask a question rather than to make a statement, the therapist might craft one without a "why" beginning. "Do we need to wear a tie today?" or "What's the dress code for today?" or "How did you decide to wear a tie today?" The therapist can save the "why" questions for those rare occasions when he or she might actually want to criticize a client's choice.[3]

## Persuasive Rhetoric

The fourth level of complexity involves the use of rhetoric as a way to expand the persuasive function of speech. A therapist cannot change a patient's undesired behavior; not by advice, not by exhortation, and not by authority. Only the patient can modify his or her own behavior. The therapist must therefore use every means available to persuade the patient to do so.

An effective tool to accomplish this goal is persuasive speech; in other words, *rhetoric*. Aristotle identified the three components of rhetoric as *Ethos*, the speaker's good character, intelligence and goodwill; *Logos*, the appeal to logic; and *Pathos*, the use of stories, metaphors and other figures of speech that appeal to a listener's emotions (Bartlett, 2019).

In the context of psychotherapy, "Ethos" is created by the therapeutic alliance that succeeds because the therapist's role as healer projects good character, intelligence and goodwill. "Logos" is supplied by the logic of the therapeutic modality selected for the treatment plan (Frank's myth and ritual) and by its particular structure and tenets (Karasu's cognitive mastery). These two components are inherent in the psychotherapy itself.

The use of "Pathos," however, is up to the therapist and requires creative initiative. In practice, this essential element includes the use of stories, anecdotes, references to well-known films, popular lyrics, television, novels, internet memes and videos, or metaphors to convey significance. It might include a joke, although humor should be used warily because it is so easily misunderstood as hurtful criticism.

Suppose a therapist wished to convey the idea that thoughtfulness in planning and careful deliberation would be useful to an impulsive patient who had difficulty seeing plans through to conclusion. One intervention might be a statement that the patient showed a pattern of thoughtlessly conceived and rarely completed plans that failed to reach their desired conclusion. This "observation" might appear to the client as a stern lecture implying a fatally flawed character rather than a helpful proposal to reach a therapy goal. A rhetorical alternative might be to use the well-known Aesop's fable of the competition between the tortoise and the hare to draw parallels with the patient's problem. The moral, "slow and steady wins the race," seems more likely to form the basis for a useful examination of the patient's difficulty and has the added benefit of being only an amusing allegory rather than a critical judgment. A shorter version of the rhetorical option would be to use the aphorism "haste makes waste" each time another instance of impulsive but ineffectual behavior arises in the therapy.[4]

## Metacommunication

The next level of complexity in communication involves the specific technique of interpersonal interaction known as metacommunication.

Therapeutic communication can operate at several levels. On the lowest level (denotation) it transmits the literal or dictionary meaning of the words. Take the statement: "My dog has fleas."

- The literal meaning is that the speaker owns a specific canine who is troubled by biting insects. The listener could respond with "I hear flea collars work well," an answer that assumes an implied request for advice.
- At the next level (connotation), the meaning can change. If the sentence is said with a laugh or with a frown or sarcastically, the meaning could be, respectively, "Everybody has problems" or "I wish I had fewer things to worry about" or "We've all got troubles and I'm no different." These implications are the metaphorical level of communication, something more implied than by the words themselves. The accompanying "data" amplifies their meaning. A direct response that understood this implied message ("I'm using the dog as an example to convey my own unhappiness") might be "I'd like to hear more about your troubles." That answer would be the standard therapist request for additional information, but does little to understand the speaker's motives.
- The third level comments on the speaker's motivation and intent. It explores the reason the statement has been made. "Are you saying your problems are trivial?" (mere fleas) or "Do you want me to feel sorry for your dog?" (and by implication, for you) or "Are we talking about your dog because you don't want to talk about your own problems?" These responses recognize the speaker's underlying meaning and focus on the purpose of the statement. Any of them would be more likely to advance therapeutic progress. "Metacommunication," as used here, applies to this third level.

The original use of the term "metacommunication" is attributed to Gregory Bateson, who defined it as "communication about communication" (Ruesch & Bateson, 1951). He observed that the words used by a speaker with their denoted meaning did not convey the entire message. The complete meaning of the words were modified and defined—connoted—by all of the additional information transmitted simultaneously by the speaker. Tone of voice, facial expressions, body language, sarcasm or irony and other non-verbal clues would tell the listener how to understand the words being spoken.[5]

For example, consider the various meanings of the words, "I'm a good person," if they are spoken with the following non-verbal additions:

- With sincerity and a smile = I'm reliable and loyal.
- With a raised voice at the end to indicate a question = you'd be wrong if you think so.
- With a frown and an angry tone = You better believe that or you're in trouble.

Thus, the same words can convey different messages, adding complexity and enrichment to any communication. Bateson understood that a therapist needed to hear the whole message to better understand the client.

A second use of the term "metacommunication" was introduced by D. J. Kiesler to describe a type of response the therapist might make to something said by a client (Kiesler, 1988). It is a communication *about* the client's statement rather than a response to it directly.

For example, consider again a client's assertion, "I'm a good person." A therapist could respond:

- To the direct content of the statement = "What makes you a good person?"
- To its implication = "You mean, you wouldn't hurt anybody?"
- To its historical context = "Did your friend simply misunderstand what you did?"

All these responses accept the content of the statement as the important part of the communication and respond directly to it in different but appropriate ways. None of these responses, however, is a metacommunication.

Now consider the following examples, again to the declaration, "I'm a good person." A therapist utilizing a metacommunicative tactic might say:

- "It sounds like you want to impress me." Or
- "Are you trying to convince yourself of that?" Or
- "What led you to tell me that at this time?"

These responses ignore the content of the statement (at least for now) and instead ask about the motivation or the timing of the client's words.

Regular communication is often compared to a tennis match: the topic alternates between the speakers with each response dependent on the previous statement.

### Example: What time is the meeting?

- It's called for nine o'clock.
- Is that AM or PM?
- The meeting is at 9:00 AM. Don't be late!

Metacommunication is like a response from the referee sitting at midcourt and judging the match. Instead of responding to the topic offered by the other speaker, the therapist comments on aspects of the communication itself.

### Example: What time is the meeting?

- Are you worried about the time?
- I don't want to be late.
- People worry too much about punctuality.

A metacommunication, then, is a response to the motivations behind a statement, the reason it was said, the impact the speaker expected from the listener. This more abstract approach considers what the communication says about the speaker's state of mind, covert agenda, or unstated feelings. When a therapist responds with a metacommunication it invites scrutiny about the purpose of the client's statement. It raises the dialogue from a mere exchange of information to a means of working on the client's problems and the goals of the therapy. As such it is an important tool, often an indispensable one, in the investigation of a critical topic.

## Modeling

The final level of communication often occurs automatically, sometimes without the therapist's conscious participation. From childhood on, people learn by first observing how others successfully function and then imitating their success through a process known as "partial identification" (Holmes, 2009). In a treatment session, the behavior of the therapist can provide a model with which the patient can identify. The ordinary behaviors therapists usually display include mature judgment, the calm consideration of the patient's difficulties leading to a set of alternatives and an understanding of antecedents and motivations. The therapist's emotional detachment from disturbing recollections and experiences the patient may recount encourages the patient to deal more successfully with those events. The therapist's confidence that difficult problems have possible solutions encourages hope and confidence in the patient. The therapist's non-judgmental attitude and positive regard for the patient may allow the patient to increase self-worth and self-esteem that in turn enhances the possibility that they can make good use of the therapy.

While it may seem that these non-verbal behaviors are a given and that therapists do not need to be explicitly aware of them, there are times when the therapist can emphasize these qualities and make better use of their effect. In particular, in dealing with clients with maladaptive personality traits—avoidant, dependent, narcissistic, obsessional and the like—the therapist who is aware of the potential for modeling adaptive behaviors can emphasize them to good effect.

To take one example: Jay Haley used to help his clients with contamination fears (an obsessive-compulsive trait) by taking off his shoe, rubbing his hand over the sole and then through his hair and across his face—all to model his indifference to possible contamination.[6]

## Summary

Communication in therapy, regardless of the methodology employed, is not the same as a social or personal discussion. The deliberate use of communicative skills allows the therapist to make efficient use of the limited time in a therapy session to achieve the maximum beneficial effect.

## Notes

1 Observer estimates of intelligence, based on auditory and visual assessment, are surprisingly accurate (Murphy et al., 2003).
2 And out of the ground the LORD GOD formed every beast of the field, and every fowl of the air, and brought *them* unto Adam to see what he would call them: and whatsoever Adam called every living creature, that *was* the name thereof. (Genesis 2:19 King James Version)
3 Not all why questions imply disapproval, of course. Some may simply request information. For example: why is the sky blue?
4 Repetitive use of the same response to each instance of a target behavior until the client is able to apply the idea unaided is an important means of "working through."
5 The absence of connotation data in texts or emails is what makes them so subject to easy misunderstanding. Emojis are an attempt to supply the missing non-verbal cues.
6 Haley demonstrated this technique at a lecture I attended. Several members of the audience squirmed and one person moaned while he did it.

## References

Bartlett, R. C. (2019). *Aristotle's art of rhetoric, translation with an interpretive essay.* University of Chicago Press.

Holmes, L. (2009). The technique of partial identification: Waking up to the world. *International Journal of Group Psychotherapy*, 59, 253–265.

Karasu, T. B. (2013). *Life witness, evolution of the psychotherapist.* Jason Aronson.

Kiesler, D. J. (1988). *Therapeutic metacommunication: Therapist impact disclosure as feedback in psychotherapy.* Consulting Psychologists Press.

Murphy, N. A., Hall, J. A., & Colvin, C. R. (2003). Accurate intelligence assessments in social interactions: Mediators and gender effects. *Journal of Personality*, 71, 465–493.

Ruesch, J., & Bateson, G. (1951). *Communication: The social matrix of psychiatry.* Norton.

Case One

# Holly

## A Troubled Teenage Marriage

### Referral

Holly applied to the mental health clinic and was evaluated by one
of the intake workers. In summary, the evaluation said:

> The patient is a 19 year old female, married six months, who
> presents with a chief complaint of "nerves."
>
> Her husband is a mechanic at an automobile dealership. She is a
> homemaker. They married one week after their high school gradu-
> ation. Alone at home she experiences nearly constant low-level
> anxiety punctuated by two or three panic attacks per day. She con-
> trols these by rebreathing into a paper bag. Her anxiety subsides
> when her husband is home. Her sleep and appetite are normal, and
> she is otherwise in good health.
>
> Mental status examination shows an alert, friendly but rest-
> less young woman with mildly pressured but goal directed
> speech. She is well groomed with somewhat heavy makeup,
> dressed in a patterned blouse and dark slacks. Memory is intact.
> Judgment is age-appropriate. Estimated IQ is 110–120. She
> denies depressed mood and suicidal ideation. There is no evi-
> dence of impaired reality testing, hallucinations or delusions.
>
> Diagnostic impression: Generalized Anxiety Disorder (F41.1)
> Plan: Individual psychotherapy

Jane had an opening in her clinic schedule. She met Holly two
weeks after her evaluation. In their initial interview, she learned
more about Holly's history:

DOI: 10.4324/9781003353003-4

## History

Holly is the youngest of three children and the only girl in an intact family. Her father is an electrician working for a medium-sized construction company. Her mother remained at home when the children were in school but has recently gone to work as an associate at the local Walmart. Holly was an anxious child who had a mild case of school phobia. In kindergarten and first grade she would cling to her mother when it was time to go to school and sometimes pretend to be sick so she could stay at home. Beginning with second grade, she gradually became more comfortable leaving home, but she never liked school, although her grades were always A's and B's. When she entered high school, she formed a close relationship with Gary, the boy who is now her husband. Gary feels she should stay at home while he supports them. She is bored at home by herself, but her friends from high school are busy with work or college and not available in the daytime. She and Gary sometimes go to parties with friends on weekends or they see her family or Gary's. He wants to start a family, but Holly does not feel ready for that. One reason she has come to the clinic is to delay the decision about getting pregnant until she has recovered from her "nerves" problem. In fact, she applied to the clinic the day after she and Gary had "a big fight" about starting a family.

## Formulation

The history and her impressions from the initial interview provide Jane with several ideas.

She conceptualizes Holly's core problem as a failure to achieve age-appropriate independence. Her history of separation anxiety in childhood, although it resolved as she grew older, nevertheless may be one foundation for her current difficulties. She is now in late adolescence, a time when peer group attachments become increasingly important and help to smooth the transition toward individuation and separation from the family. Because she is married and at home, she has hardly any contact with her school friends. Her marriage to her high school boyfriend immediately after graduation suggests she was unable to face the future on her own. Her opposition to Gary's plan for her immediate pregnancy is a hopeful sign that she recognizes that she is not ready for this step and that she can assert some independence in the marriage. To the extent that she bases her resistance to getting pregnant on her "nerves," however, suggests that she cannot fully take responsibility for her decision, and it raises the problem of secondary gain: that she will resist her "nerves" getting better because she needs the illness to justify her stance. Her motivation for therapy is high. Her motivation for change is moderate.

Using these ideas, Jane can formulate Holly's case: She is a 19-year-old, recently married woman with generalized anxiety and panic episodes who is facing a developmental challenge in the transition from adolescence to young adult. She may be predisposed to this stalemate *because* of early difficulties with separation and individuation.[1] She is socially isolated *because* her marriage choice has precluded the usual developmental steps of higher education or entrance into the job market. Her isolation at home appears to fuel her general anxiety *because* she lacks social and friendship supports. Her early marriage may represent an attempt to avoid adult independence *because* her husband appears to have the dominant "parental" role as breadwinner and decision-maker in the relationship.

(Formulation Category: Developmental)[2]

## Treatment Plan

Based on her formulation, Jane created a treatment plan. The AIM of her proposed therapy can be summarized as "develop more adult independence" and may be achieved through two therapy GOALS:

- Achieve more adult independence from her family of origin by advancing the normal separation required when an individual establishes a family of procreation.
- Establish a more independent role in the marriage.

Jane's judgment of Holly's suitability for psychotherapy places her in the moderate range: she is neither intellectually challenged nor overly intellectualized. Her emotional intelligence and her capacity to form an alliance with the therapist both appear adequate. She seems average or above in her capacity to handle abstract ideas and to modify her behavior. For these reasons, Jane decides to employ two STRATEGIES. Primarily, she will use a psychodynamic approach to help Holly reach these goals, one that will include identification of the key problems, confronting Holly with the areas that need change, interpreting the reasons for the developmental delay, and helping her work through the changes needed. Some cognitive-behavioral work may be needed for the anxiety problem.

When Jane discusses this plan with her, Holly accepts her proposal but she also wants the therapy to help her overcome the anxiety ("nerves") that brought her to the clinic, and Jane agrees that this third goal is important as well. This discussion results in a therapeutic contract based on weekly sessions.

The following session is the first "therapy session" after the initial evaluation. The 45-minute appointment is scheduled for 9:00 AM at the mental health clinic. In this early meeting, Jane hopes to accomplish three things. She wants to strengthen the therapeutic alliance. Holly's hopeful expectation that the treatment will be helpful and her trust in and reliance on Jane are nonspecific factors that will support and enhance the work of the therapy. She needs to establish a working template that will carry over into future sessions. Whatever type of psychotherapy is employed, the early work must include some education and "training" that will help the patient understand what is required if the treatment is to succeed. She expects to initiate work on the major therapeutic objectives to help Holly move toward more independence from her family and within the marriage.

## SESSION TWO

A Tuesday morning. The mental health clinic is in a low brick building surrounded by an open-air parking lot. Holly enters a main reception area where she checks in at reception and she is then directed down a short hallway to a smaller waiting area, a window-less room with gray carpeting, vinyl-upholstered armchairs and a low table with a few magazines. A small television set high on one wall is tuned to a local cable news station. Three office doors open off the waiting area.

At 9:00 AM, Jane opens one of the office doors. She wears an ivory blouse and dark gray skirt with low-heeled shoes. She has on a beaded necklace and wears a dark blue, open cardigan over the blouse.

Holly smiles and gets up to come into the office. The clinic office is a square room, about 12 feet on a side, furnished with three upholstered chairs. The two set on either side of a small table that holds a lamp and a box of tissues are the client chairs and the third, Jane's chair, is also next to a small side table, facing them. The floor is covered in dark green carpeting; the walls are white and bare. A large window with a half-opened blind lets in some light, but the main illumination is a fluorescent ceiling fixture.

Time remaining
45 minutes

| Jane | Good morning. |
|------|---------------|

*Jane begins with a short, neutral social greeting. She wants to avoid setting up any prolonged opening ritual, such as a discussion of the weather or current events or even a "how are you," that would use up therapy time or distort the working atmosphere of the session.*

*Jane notes that Holly is dressed appropriately in a simple top, jeans and flats. Her cell phone is stuck in the back pocket of her jeans. She carries a black handbag. Her makeup seems a bit heavy for an early morning appointment: eyeshadow, mascara, a dark red lipstick. She looks a little tense and perhaps a bit excited.*

*Jane takes her chair. She sits comfortably against the chair back with her hands folded in her lap and her feet on the floor, a position that conveys an open, attentive attitude.*

Holly          (Smiles) Hi.

Jane           How did you feel this week? How was your anxiety?

               *Holly sits halfway back on the chair cushion,*
               *with her arms across her stomach and feet*
               *pulled back with ankles crossed. Her body*
               *language conveys tense and defensive. Jane*
               *introduces a NAME for Holly's "nerves."*
               *She wants Holly to think of the problem as*
               *psychological and specific rather than vague*
               *and physical.*

Holly          Not too bad. It's mostly first thing in the morning, after
               Gary leaves for work. Once I get started on the house-
               work and get busy it kind of takes my mind off it.

Jane           (Nods) So things are a little better.

               *Holly originally presented with nearly*
               *constant anxiety and occasional panic, yet*
               *she now reports significant reductions in both*
               *its frequency and intensity despite the absence*
               *of any therapy directed at this symptom.*
               *Her improvement may represent a PLACEBO*
               *EFFECT or it could reflect an expectation that*
               *Jane will "shield" her from whatever the*
               *cause of this symptom may turn out to be,*
               *an early TRANSFERENCE phenomenon. Her*
               *explanation that keeping busy is responsible*
               *could lead to a discussion of distraction as a*
               *coping mechanism and of various ways to use*
               *it to control her "nerves," but Jane does not*
               *plan to use that approach.*

               *Of the three GOALS in the plan, anxiety*
               *reduction was the one most important to*
               *Holly, so Jane decides to focus on it first. Her*
               *attention to Holly's main concern will help*

> *to strengthen the* THERAPEUTIC ALLIANCE. *Her question asks for a simple historical report and should be non-threatening.*

Holly   (Shrugs) I think so.

Jane   So you're not anxious when Gary's home?

> *Jane chooses to concentrate on the connection between the anxiety and Gary's departure, with the* HYPOTHESIS *that it is the stimulus for a kind of reverse separation anxiety. Her* IDENTIFICATION[3] *is the first step in the psychodynamic sequence.*

Holly   No, I'm thinking about getting his breakfast and stuff like that. (She uncrosses her arms and rests them on the arms of the chair)

Jane   So, just to be clear, then: you don't feel anxious from the time you wake up in the morning until Gary leaves the house. Is that right?

> *Jane notes that Holly relaxes a bit and looks less defensive.* CLARIFICATION *of her observation is the second step.*

Holly   That's right. Well, I know he's going to leave, so I do start to worry when it gets to be time for him to go to work.

Jane   And then what happens? After he leaves.

> *The* CLARIFICATION *has elicited some new information. Jane wants to explore it further.*

Holly   (Frowns) Well, once he's out the door I feel uneasy. You know, with the whole day ahead of me. Then I think about what I have to do. Clean up from breakfast.

Maybe get the laundry together. It depends. If I can get my mind on other things it usually helps.

Jane    So at that point you're still feeling in control. You're not anxious.

*This statement introduces the idea that "control" would be a helpful tool Holly might use to reduce her anxiety. She also repeats the NAME (anxious) to reinforce a term that she hopes will give Holly a new way to think about her problem.*

Holly    (Shakes her head) Not then. I guess it's when I stop and take a break. Like, I'll have a cup of coffee, put on some music, watch TV. Then I start to feel restless and pretty soon my nerves are bothering me again.

Jane    Does that happen on a weekend? When Gary's not working?

*Holly ignores Jane's suggestion that loss of control makes her anxious and continues to use her term, "nerves." Jane has raised the idea as a statement rather than as a question and does not have enough evidence to know if Holly resists the idea or if it is simply off the mark. She broadens the discussion, indirectly, by the focus on another time Gary would be home.*

Holly    No, not if we're busy.

Jane    You think that's it? Keeping busy prevents your nerves?

*Jane offers a mild challenge to Holly's idea using Holly's own word in order to sharpen her CONFRONTATION and to lay the groundwork for a later INTERPRETATION.*

Holly        (Cocks her head) Well, yeah. Don't you think so?

Jane         I think that could be part of it. The other part might be
             that when Gary's there your anxiety's okay.

> *Asking what Jane thinks may indicate
> that Holly sees her as the expert and the
> authority who will give her the answers
> to her problems. Her expectation might
> lead to a problem later, as she waited to
> hear "the answer" from Jane instead of
> sharing in a collaborative effort to solve
> her problems. Jane does not challenge
> this idea now because she wants to move
> toward further examination of the source
> of Holly's anxiety.*
>
> *Jane could duck the question and ask Holly
> what she thinks, inviting her to be more
> introspective and more responsible for her
> own recovery, but if she took that path it
> would divert the inquiry into a "process"
> discussion. At this stage of the treatment
> Jane is willing to take a more active role in
> the interest of moving the therapy forward.
> She therefore acknowledges Holly's notion
> but then suggests the alternative idea she
> wants her to think about.*

Holly        (Sounding a bit testy) I like it when he's around,
             obviously. He's my husband.

                                              Time remaining
                                              35 minutes

Jane         Could he also be a kind of security blanket?

> *Holly's irritation reflects her RESISTANCE to
> this idea. Jane counters by now offering the
> INTERPRETATION for which she has been laying*

*a FOUNDATION. She takes a risk in making an early interpretation (carefully putting it in the form of a question) because her ALLIANCE with Holly may not be strong enough and because she still knows relatively little about Holly and her problems. It contains only a mild suggestion that dependency problems might play a role in Holly's anxiety. It follows a tried-and-true therapy maxim; namely, "stay on the surface," and avoids the more upsetting implication that Gary could serve as a parent substitute.*

Holly        (Scrunches her face as if smelling something unpleasant) You mean like Linus in the Peanuts cartoons? That would be kind of pathetic. You think I'm being a baby?

Jane        (Remains silent)

*Holly's initial response is to be mildly outraged and insulted, perhaps as a way to reject the INTERPRETATION. Although Holly's last comment raises a possible TRANSFERENCE issue and could undermine the THERAPEUTIC ALLIANCE, Jane wants to wait and see what Holly's full response to her interpretation might be.*

Holly        (After the silence builds for almost a minute) Okay, I suppose I do feel better when he's around. I mean, he'd be there if anything happened.

Jane        Like what?

*In order to deal with this new, more subtle, disagreement with Jane's interpretation, she asks Holly for details.*

Holly      (Looks distressed) Like... I don't know. If I passed out or I had a heart attack or something.

Jane       (Maintains a neutral emphasis in her voice) A heart attack?

> *Jane responds to the emotional intensity of Holly's statement by "asking" about the topic. She does not want to sound skeptical or dismissive. At age 19, Holly's fear seems, at this point, to be exaggerated.*

Holly      That's what it feels like sometimes. My heart starts pounding and I feel light-headed.

Jane       (Still keeps her voice neutral) Do you have any history of heart problems?

> *Holly appears to be describing a panic attack rather than the constant anxiety that Jane thought they were discussing. Perhaps Holly is revealing an anticipatory anxiety related to the panic rather than generalized anxiety. Jane notes that the discussion is veering away from her INTERPRETATION, an indication of RESISTANCE, but she chooses not to confront Holly on the diversion at this early stage, especially because control of the anxiety is one of the therapy GOALS. Jane avoids any response that Holly could experience as pooh-poohing her worry and instead asks about evidence for the fear.*

Holly      No, but you never know. A boy in my school died during football practice. He had something wrong with his heart that nobody knew about.

| | |
|---|---|
| Jane | I see. Have you done anything about this worry? Seen a heart doctor, for instance? |

*Holly reveals a "realistic" source of her worry. Her health fears may be another expression of her general anxiety. The discussion is now far away from the loaded topic of Gary as a security blanket. Jane wants to explore the possibility of an additional problem: HYPOCHONDRIASIS.*

| | |
|---|---|
| Holly | No. Do you think I should? |
| Jane | That's up to you. |

*She rejects Holly's child-like need to ask Jane to make the decision for her.*

| | |
|---|---|
| Holly | Yes, but what's your advice? |
| Jane | I don't give advice. |

*Jane decides to confront this dependence issue now before it becomes a bigger problem.*

| | |
|---|---|
| Holly | (Looks hurt) So, what, you just don't care? |
| Jane | What makes you think that? |

*Jane narrowly avoids a why question ("Why do you think that?"). Once again, a TRANSFERENCE issue distorts the discussion. Evidently, Holly's defense when rejected is to try to evoke guilt. Uncertain if it needs to be dealt with at this early stage, Jane uses a METACOMMUNICATION to ask her for the evidence for her conclusion.*

| | |
|---|---|
| Holly | It's obvious. If you cared what happened to me, you'd at least give me your opinion. |
| Jane | Is there any other reason you think I don't care? |

*Again, checking whether Holly has any other unexpressed basis for her concern.*

| | |
|---|---|
| Holly | (With raised eyebrows) Isn't that enough? |

Time remaining
25 minutes

| | |
|---|---|
| Jane | Hmm. Here's an alternative idea: if I told you what to do, it could undermine our work together. Instead of the two of us figuring out what's wrong and how to fix it, you'd leave it all to me and assume I had all the answers. I'd be responsible for your recovery and you'd be off the hook. You wouldn't have to take any responsibility for yourself. A few minutes ago, you asked if I thought you were a baby. If I told you what to do, I really would be treating you like a baby, wouldn't I? |

*Rather than attempting to further explore the TRANSFERENCE or to leap into an INTERPRETATION, Jane chooses to speak to Holly's "adult" self, drawing on the REAL RELATIONSHIP, and to educate her about an underlying principle of their therapy together.*

| | |
|---|---|
| Holly | (Holly sits back and fold her arms across her chest) I guess so. |
| Jane | It's frustrating, I know. |

*With this METACOMMUNICATION, Jane acknowledges Holly's feeling in hopes to repair the damage to the THERAPEUTIC ALLIANCE.*

> *Jane is aware of the high dropout rate early in therapy and wants to mend anything that frays the alliance before it causes a breach.*

Holly   No, it's all right. I understand. (Her eyes have filled with tears and she avoids eye contact, looking over Jane's shoulder. Jane is silent and waits for her to resume) So, anyway, that's why I feel better if Gary's around. (After another pause) Is that it for today?

Jane   We have some time yet.

> *Apparently one of Holly's defensive maneuvers is to leave the field when she is frustrated and disappointed. Jane hesitates to attack the defense because Holly is already distressed, and the THERAPEUTIC ALLIANCE has been weakened, so she simply makes a realistic observation.*

Holly   Okay. (After saying this, Holly sinks back against the chair, crosses her arms over her chest, and remains silent)

Jane   (Sits through some non-verbal minutes) When you were in high school did you ever get a detention?

> *The session has reached a "flexion point." Holly's withdrawal into silence is a form of RESISTANCE that blocks further progress in the session. Jane could assume a passive stance and remain silent herself, letting the tension build. She could offer a METACOMMUNICATION; for example, that Holly appears to be angry with her and invite her to put her feelings into words.*

*She could label Holly's behavior as "pouting like an angry child," resuming the discussion of "being a baby." She could again discuss how her refusal to give Holly advice helps the therapy effort or she could raise a new topic, taking more responsibility for the management of the session but ignoring the silence-as-resistance problem. Each of these choices might be appropriate in a particular therapy approach, and would lay the groundwork for how Jane handles future episodes of RESISTANCE.*

*Jane waits long enough to determine that Holly is unlikely to break the silence. She is inclined to take a more active role in the therapy, in part because of her own personality (she is often impatient with slow progress or roadblocks) and in part because she recognizes that Holly, still an adolescent, will not respond well to what she will see as a battle of wills. Her question is based on the recognition that this young woman is barely out of high school, and Holly's passive-aggressive, I'll-just-wait-it-out body language reminds her of a student forced to stay after class. The seemingly "out of the blue" question LAYS A FOUNDATION for Jane's subsequent comment.*

Holly         (Reluctantly) No. Why?

Jane          Sitting there like that, you look like someone just waiting for her punishment to end.

              *She RENAMES Holly's disappointment as "punishment" to underline the inappropriate and exaggerated nature of her response to Jane's stance on "advice."*

Holly   (Sighs, loudly, and rolls her eyes)

Jane   The idea in therapy is to put your feelings into words. That way you and I can figure out what the problems are and how to deal with them. Do you think you can do that now? Put how you're feeling **right now** into words?

*Building again on the REAL RELATIONSHIP, Jane makes an effort again to educate Holly.*

Holly   I'm… annoyed.

Jane   Annoyed with me?

*This euphemism for feeling angry is better than no response at all and shows Holly remains accessible.*

*Jane emphasizes that Holly's anger is with her, not some abstract idea or general concept. She wants to establish that a relationship problem has arisen and to help Holly confront her about it.*

Holly   (Shrugs, her expression more discouraged than angry) This isn't going how I thought it would.

Jane   How did you think it would go?

*Holly appears to question the THERAPEUTIC CONTRACT, raising a "red flag" that Jane must immediately address and deal with to prevent both a rupture in the THERAPEUTIC*

*ALLIANCE and a possible impending*
*STRUCTURAL IMPASSE.*

Holly

(Shakes her head) I don't know. I thought you'd be able to tell me what to do. You're supposed to be the expert here. If I could figure things out on my own I wouldn't need you, would I?

Jane

You're raising some good points. Let me try to give you some answers. First of all, I am an expert... in psychotherapy. I'm not an expert in you. I haven't known you very long and, so far, I don't know a lot about you. So, if you think about it, the only expert on you is: you. We need to work together to combine my therapy skills with your knowledge of yourself, **your** background, **your** feelings, the things only you can know about, so that I can help you figure things out on your own. My job is to listen to what you tell me about yourself and put it together in a way that helps you understand your problems and to make the changes you need for things to get better for you. If we can do that, then by the end you won't need me anymore.

> *The emergence of Holly's assumption that she would be the passive recipient of an expert's ministrations shows the early emergence of a "parental" TRANSFERENCE, not unexpected in an adolescent. It is an advantageous admission, however, that allows Jane to deal with this fantasy in a helpful way.*
>
> *Again, Jane opts for an educational response and ignores the early TRANSFERENCE feelings. Holly has only recently emerged from childhood dependence, on both her family and her teachers, so it is less*

*surprising that her naïve expectation is for
the therapist to be an authority who directs
her. By adopting a didactic stance, she is,
in effect, using this expectation to advance
the therapy work. She attempts to "direct"
her toward collaboration in the therapy, a
type of PARADOXICAL INTERVENTION. (When
she says "I won't tell you what to do," she
is simultaneously saying, "I'm telling you
what to do.") Finally, she foreshadows the
termination of the therapy. At the moment,
that idea may seem attractive to Holly, but,
if things go well, chances are she won't want
therapy to end when the time comes.*

Holly        So if I'm the expert, what am I supposed to do?

Time remaining
15 minutes

Jane         Exactly what you've been doing: tell me about your-
             self, what your life has been like, how you feel about
             things, your relationships with the other people in
             your life.

             *Holly has made another request for advice,
             but this time for guidance in the therapy
             process. Jane is willing to provide this
             guidance as part of her educational effort.*

Holly        Okay. (Pause) I don't know where to start.

Jane         Hmm. Could you tell me more about your family?

             *Since Jane's HYPOTHESIS is that Holly
             has been overly dependent on and unable
             to separate from her family, she doesn't*

*mind, in this early session, asking for more family history.*

Holly    Well, my father's kind of old-fashioned. He didn't want my Mom to work when we were growing up and I don't think he's that happy about it now that she's got a job.

Jane    Gary's the same way, isn't he?

*Holly's choice of this topic provides an unexpected opening to explore her choice of a husband and Jane decides to pursue it rather than asking for more history.*

Holly    I'm not raising any kids. I don't have to be home.

Jane    And yet you are.

*Jane lays a FOUNDATION for the HYPOTHESIS that the parallel between Holly's father and her choice of husband may contribute to her current predicament.*

Holly    Yeah, but only because of my nerves.

Jane    If you didn't have the anxiety, you'd get a job?

*Once again, Jane carefully RENAMES the "nerves" as anxiety, a defined symptom. Up to now, however, Holly has not accepted the substitution.*

Holly    Maybe. If Gary'd let me.

Jane    (With raised eyebrows and a skeptical expression) If he'd "**let**" you?"

> *By this somewhat exaggerated response Jane attempts to both identify an important issue (developing independence in the marriage) and to confront Holly with the way her attitude underpins her over-dependence on Gary. This simple TACTIC, reflecting Holly's words with a change of emphasis, could prove to be the most important therapeutic intervention of the session.*

Holly   That sounds bad, doesn't it?

Jane    (Remains silent)

Holly   I dunno. He feels pretty strongly about it. He's the breadwinner, I'm the housewife.

Jane    Like your parents.

> *Since Holly has characterized her parent's relationship as "old-fashioned," Jane wants to indirectly REFRAME her relationship with Gary as equally unsatisfactory.*

Holly   Yeah. My Mom was never that okay with it. She's much happier now that she's got that crummy job at Walmart. Funny, huh?

Jane    (Remains silent)

> *And so does Holly, but this time her silence appears to result from her thinking over what has been said in the last few minutes. Because "the wheels are turning," Jane does not attempt to re-engage her as she did earlier.*

| Holly | Gary's idea is that I take care of the house, keep it clean, cook the meals and all that stuff. That's what I'm used to. That's what my house was like when I was growing up. And I go along with it. It's what I expected. |
|---|---|
| Jane | But you said your Mom was unhappy. |

*Since Holly refers to her mother as "Mom," Jane uses the same word, matching her DICTION to Holly's.*

| Holly | Yeah, she was. |
|---|---|
| Jane | So, are you unhappy, too? |

*She wants to strengthen the INTERPRETATION.*

| Holly | I didn't think so. I mean, I like it when the house is clean. I like to cook. |
|---|---|
| Jane | You said earlier that you're okay in the morning when Gary's home and you're still okay while you do the household chores, but after that is when you start to feel anxious. |

*Holly seems to back away from the implication that if she is as unhappy as her mother she might look for the same solution; namely, to defy Gary and strike out on her own.*

*Jane reminds Holly of their earlier discussion about Gary as her security blanket.*

| Holly | Yeah. |
|---|---|
| Jane | What's going through your mind at that point? Gary leaves, the housework is done, and then what happens? |

*She asks for Holly's* AFFECTIVE EXPERIENCE
*to being left alone.*

Holly        (Looks puzzled) I don't know.

Jane         Okay, well, let's start with when Gary leaves. What
             happens then? Does he just walk out the door? Do
             you say anything? How does that work?

             *Jane hopes a focus on specific details will
             evoke more useful material than has been
             produced by the more general discussion
             so far.*

Holly        Um, after he finishes breakfast he usually goes to the
             bathroom. Then he comes out, gets his coat, kisses
             me goodbye and goes out to his truck.

Jane         So, he's in the bathroom and you're waiting for him
             to come out and leave. How do you feel then?

             *Jane looks for the emotional content, the*
             AFFECTIVE EXPERIENCE *of this crucial moment
             in Holly's day.*

Holly        I'm a little nervous. I know he's leaving, so I'm going
             to be by myself all day. He won't be back until the
             end of the day and I'm on my own all that time.

                                              Time remaining
                                              5 minutes

Jane         And then he does leave.

             *A* FOUNDATION *statement.*

Holly        Yeah.

Jane         How do you feel at that moment?

*Emphasizing again the focus on emotion.*

Holly      Sad. And a little like I'm... I don't know. We used
           to have a dog when I was a kid and when she was
           a puppy and we'd leave her in the house she would
           whine and cry and act like she wouldn't ever see us
           again. I guess I feel a little like that, too.

Jane       Abandoned.

           *Jane supplies the NAME for the feeling that
           Holly could only describe by her anecdote.
           Given Holly's history of school phobia and
           separation anxiety, the word, abandoned,
           encapsulates a complex set of emotions and
           experiences that could be important in future
           sessions.*

Holly      Yeah. (She starts to cry. Then, wiping her eyes:) Oh,
           this is stupid.

Jane       It's not stupid if that's how you feel.

           *The force of Jane's relabeling Holly's
           feeling as "abandoned" elicits a strong
           affective response, confirming its
           authenticity. By validating Holly's response
           Jane not only encourages her to accept her
           feelings but also tries to empower her and
           increase her self-esteem.*

Holly      (Continues to cry) But I shouldn't feel that way.

Jane       That's something we should talk more about, but our
           time is up for today and we have to stop.

           *The time is 9:45 AM. Jane resists the tempta-
           tion to extend the session because Holly is
           crying and because she is dealing with an*

*important issue. That would set a bad prec-
edent, not only because it would encourage
Holly to wait to bring up difficult issues and
emotions as the session neared its end—in
order to assure that she can escape from them
and, perhaps as well, to delay the separation
from her therapist—but also because it would
suggest that dealing with an emotional subject
is extraordinary rather than the usual and
expected type of material the therapy should
deal with. She uses a formulaic expression
("our time is up and we have to stop") to
signal the end of the available time, a phrase
she will use to conclude every session as a
small ritual that will make it easier for Holly
to accept the end of their contact for that day.*

Holly          (Takes a tissue from the box on the table at her side
               and dries her tears) Okay. I'll see you next week.

(Jane stands up and Holly also stands and walks to the door without
looking at Jane. Holly leaves.)

### Discussion

How well did Jane accomplish what she wanted to do in this first
session? Her first objective was to strengthen the therapeutic alliance. While it prevailed in general, the alliance was actually threatened at two points in the session, the first only mildly but more
seriously later.

The first challenge was Jane's interpretation that Gary served as
a "security blanket." The idea that Holly is acting (in her words)
"like a baby" is a narcissistic blow, especially to someone in late
adolescence who hopes she has left her childhood behind and wants
to see herself as an adult. In general, an accurate interpretation tends
to undermine the alliance because it disturbs the patient's internal
mental stability. The impulse to protect against this "assault" may

be projected onto the therapist, the "attacker." The patient can recognize the validity of the interpretation and at the same time resist the need to confront it and resent the person who offers it.[4]

The second challenge arose when Jane flatly stated that she would not offer advice. Holly's response was, "you don't care about me." Her disappointment had a more serious impact on the therapeutic alliance since it was based on a fantasy, the transference perception that Jane was a protective parent. Jane's educational response appeared to be only partially, and probably temporarily, successful, and she should expect that the issue will arise again in future discussions.

The alliance survived these two setbacks. One can think of the alliance as a kind of "therapeutic bank account" in which the therapist stores up trust and acceptance. Asking the patient to face something uncomfortable or threatening "spends" some of this accumulated capital. It may need to build up again before making the next effort to challenge the patient to modify troublesome behaviors. Jane did not appear to strengthen the alliance, but neither did she permanently damage it.

Her second objective was to establish a working template for the combined use of directive and exploratory therapeutic strategies. Jane used some direction throughout the session: She began the session by asking Holly about her anxiety symptoms during the prior week rather than waiting for Holly to pick a topic or asking an open-ended question, such as "what's on your mind today?" She offered Holly several educational "instructions" at points of difficulty within the session. She asked for particular items of history; for example, when she questioned Holly on the specifics of Gary's departure in the mornings.

She also employed psychodynamic procedures: She made judicious use of silence to encourage Holly to provide therapeutic material. She identified problem areas and tried to clarify exactly what was involved. She offered a significant interpretation (the security blanket) and had a second opportunity to begin the process of working through. She offered an indirect interpretation when she labeled Holly's response to Gary's leaving for work as her feeling "abandoned."

Jane's choice of this combination reflects her own preferences and training, but it also fits with her patient's needs. The adolescent brain is not fully developed. Even in the late teens and early twenties, judgment remains impulsive and immature and the capacity for abstract thought is incomplete. These factors make it more difficult for patients in this age group to handle prolonged silence and passivity that might be better tolerated with older patients. Adolescents usually do better with a therapist who is more actively engaged.

Jane's third objective was to begin work on Holly's need to separate from her family of origin and to be more independent in the marriage. Jane made a reasonable start on these goals. She confronted Holly's expectation that Gary controlled what Holly could do when she challenged Holly's statement, "...if Gary'd let me." She began to develop the parallel between Holly's role expectations in the marriage and her mother's unhappy role in her family of origin. Jane made no specific effort to raise Holly's need to separate further from her family, but the discussion of her father's authoritarian, "old fashioned" behavior, her mother's unhappiness with her own dependence, and her mother's delight when she finally got a job, all laid the groundwork for later work on this issue.

In summary, this first therapy session after the clinic intake and Jane's initial meeting was a successful effort to initiate the therapeutic process.

## SESSION THREE

Another Tuesday morning appointment, one week later. Holly has arrived at the clinic 20 minutes early and paced for a few minutes in the small waiting room before settling into one of the chairs. She wears a dark red T-shirt with jeans and boots. The heavy eye makeup is missing but she wears dark red lipstick. Jane arrives a few minutes later. She nods to Holly and tells her she'll be with her in a few minutes. She enters the office and closes the door. Despite

Holly's early arrival, she waits until 9:00 AM and then opens the office door. Holly enters and flops into the chair. Jane takes her seat.

Time remaining
45 minutes

Holly            (Leaning forward) Gary and I had a big fight!

Jane             (Raises her eyebrows) When was this?

> *An intercurrent event can be a distraction or an opportunity. Jane's question acknowledges the topic and invites Holly to give an account of the "big fight," beginning with how recent it was, and therefore how vivid are the feelings it aroused.*

Holly            (Speaks in a pressured, loud whisper) Last night. I told him I was coming here this morning and he asked me if I really needed it and I said I did and he said, "for what?" So I told him I was trying to figure some things out, like whether I should get out of the house and get a job and earn some money. And he said, "Where'd **that** come from?" So I told him from you and he got mad and said it was none of your business, or something like that, and I should quit coming here if that's the kind of shit you were telling me. And then it went on from there and I ended up sleeping on the couch in front of the TV and this morning he just got dressed and went off to work. He didn't even stay for breakfast.

Jane             Sounds like you're still angry about it.

> *Holly's whispering suggests she wants to keep this news between Jane and herself. In fact, it reminds Jane of the sharing of secrets common among high school girls.*

*She elects not to comment on this odd
presentation because the content of Holly's
account is more important than how she
delivers it. The episode immediately pre-
ceded today's appointment and, in fact,
was provoked by it, so it is both fresh and,
to Holly, urgent. It raises a challenge to
the therapy itself, since Gary seems to feel
threatened by Holly's attendance and wants
her to quit, a compelling reason to deal
with it immediately. Jane temporizes with
a METACOMMUNICATION that comments on
Holly's affect rather than the substance of
the event, hoping to elicit further details.*

Holly        (Shrugs) I guess.

Jane         And how did you feel when he left for work without
             breakfast?

             *Since Holly doesn't add to her report, she
             returns to the crucial moment they identified
             in the prior session, when Holly feels "aban-
             doned" and anxious.*

Holly        I was still kind of annoyed. I'm not going to stop
             coming just because he gets pissed.

Jane         So, annoyed, but no anxiety?

             *Holly's response suggests that the
             THERAPEUTIC ALLIANCE is intact. She has not
             wavered in her determination to continue
             therapy, nor has Gary's behavior raised
             doubts about its benefits. Jane emphasizes
             the importance of this change in Holly's
             handling of this critical moment by
             underlining the absence of her anxiety.*

Holly    No. (Grins) How about that!

Jane    Pretty impressive.

> *This praise may prove to be injudicious. On the one hand, it reinforces a behavior that is consistent with the therapy* GOAL *of more autonomy in the marriage. On the other, it undermines Holly's achievement if it suggests that she acted to get Jane's approval rather than for her own self-respect. The risk is greater because, in the argument with Gary, she cited Jane as the authority for the idea of getting a job. A more subtle, and more significant, risk is that Holly may interpret the praise as Jane's opposition to the marriage, rather than merely her approval of tolerating Gary's departure without feeling abandoned and anxious. A better* METACOMMUNICATIVE *response may have been, "You feel good about it," because it would acknowledge Holly's recognition of her own success.*

Holly    So, what do I do now?

Jane    What do you want to do?

> *After taking a step toward independence, Holly now feels less certain. Once again, she seeks Jane's advice, reflecting her problem with self-sufficiency. Jane does not explain again that she does not give advice, since the more important topic here is Holly's next step with Gary. Instead, she simply turns the question back to Holly.*

Holly    I don't know. I don't want to stop coming here and I don't want him telling me what I can and can't do, but I don't want him angry at me either.

| | |
|---|---|
| Jane | That's a lot of "don't wants." What is it that you do want? |

*Her comment implies that Holly is in charge of her own life. Indirectly, she supports Holly's empowerment as an independent person, not merely an extension of her husband.*

| | |
|---|---|
| Holly | (Giggles) That's funny. People don't usually ask me what I want. (Leans back in the chair) I guess I'd like a little respect. Maybe I'm not the person Gary thinks I am. |

| | |
|---|---|
| Jane | The happy little housewife? |

*This image, a use of RHETORIC, offers the INTERPRETIVE hint that a subservient role is undesirable.*

| | |
|---|---|
| Holly | Yeah. Like my mother was. |

| | |
|---|---|
| Jane | But she wasn't so happy, was she? |

*Holly's IDENTIFICATION with her mother may help her follow the same path toward independence.*

| | |
|---|---|
| Holly | No. (Pauses) Well, I could talk to my Mom about getting a job at Walmart. Maybe part-time, at least to start. (Frowns) But how would I get there? I don't have a car and Gary takes the truck every day. And if I even tried to get a job, Gary'd go ape-shit. I know he would. |

Time remaining
35 minutes

| | |
|---|---|
| Jane | Are you afraid of him? |

*Jane focuses on the relationship problem rather than the mechanics of job-seeking.*

*She does not suggest, for example, that
Holly could look for a job within walking
distance of her home, or on a bus line, or
even exploring getting her own vehicle.
Driving and car ownership are common
steps toward, and markers of, adulthood,
ideas that may be helpful to introduce at a
later time.*

| | |
|---|---|
| Holly | No! (Frowns) Well, maybe a little. I don't want him to be mad at me all the time. |
| Jane | Because...? |

*Although it is only a one-word question, this
response could be an important intervention.
By not accepting her statement at face value,
Jane suggests Holly could tolerate Gary's
anger in the service of the more important
issue of her greater autonomy.*

| | |
|---|---|
| Holly | Because it makes me feel bad. Because he walked out this morning. Because he might leave and not come back. |
| Jane | So if he doesn't get his way, he'll divorce you? |

*Holly CATASTROPHIZES a disagreement into a
threat to the marriage. Jane wants to challenge this NEGATIVE OVERGENERALIZATION.
She begins by restating it so Holly hears
more clearly what she is saying.*

| | |
|---|---|
| Holly | Maybe not divorce, but he might go stay with one of his friends. |
| Jane | So, a separation, then? Even that sounds a bit extreme. Has he ever done that before? |

*She again challenges the OVERGENERALIZA-*
*TION by asking for specifics.*

Holly        No. But we didn't have a fight like this before.

Jane         You've been married how long?

*This question, to which Jane already knows*
*the answer, LAYS A FOUNDATION to challenge*
*Holly's implication that their argument was*
*unique and is preparation to challenge this*
*OVERGENERALIZATION.*

Holly        Six months. But we started going out in ninth grade.

Jane         Ninth grade. So that's, what, five years that you're
             together? And you must have had some fights in all
             that time. Did he ever break up with you?

*Jane gathers more details to challenge the*
*generalization.*

Holly        Well, no.

Jane         So let's see what you're saying: Gary would give
             up on the marriage after only six months because
             you and he disagreed on whether you should get
             a job. That's all it would take? One fight and he
             gives up?

*Jane makes Holly's fear concrete as a way*
*to show it is an extreme explanation.*

Holly        I guess not. (Sighs) I hope not.

Jane         And suppose he did. Left you and stayed somewhere
             else. Wouldn't that suggest he cared more about him-
             self and what he thinks a marriage should be than
             about you and what would make you happy?

*Jane subtly MODELS a more independent stance
with the implication that these ideas are what
Jane herself would feel, inviting a PARTIAL
IDENTIFICATION. With this remark, Jane not
only continues to confront the OVERGENERALI-
ZATION but also suggests a possible stance for
Holly to take in the ongoing conflict. Again,
there is a risk that Jane could allow her own
opinion to influence Holly's behavior.*

Holly        (Tentatively) Yeah, maybe.

Jane        Sometimes one of the partners in a marriage can use
anger and intimidation to control the other.

*A NORMATIVE statement and a generalization
with the risk of unintended consequences.
Jane labels Gary's behavior in a negative
way, suggesting that he can be over-con-
trolling, although she has no real evidence
yet that he is. On the one hand, this stance
suggests that she is strongly on Holly's side,
a position that may help the THERAPEUTIC
ALLIANCE. On the other hand, she may be
fomenting discontent in the couple's relationship with future adverse consequences.
Breaking them up is not one of the therapy
GOALS. A more useful approach might be to
explore Holly's feelings when confronted
with Gary's anger: if she felt intimidated, the
question of Gary's intention to control her
could be raised in a more targeted way.*

Holly        Really? You think that's what he's doing?

Jane        I don't know. What do you think?

*Jane implies Holly is the expert, not her.*

Holly        (Thoughtfully) Maybe.

Jane         Well, of course, I don't know Gary. I don't really
             know whether that's the way he is. So, let's go back
             to the question of whether you should go out to work.

             *Jane sees this aspect of the discussion is prob-*
             *lematic and tries to return to the more straight-*
             *forward issue of Holly's independence.*

Holly        I want to, but I don't know if I can. And I guess
             Gary's gonna come home tonight and then what?
             What if he's cooled off? Should I bring it up again?

Jane         Sounds like you're still worried about his anger. Do
             you think he might be worried about you? You were
             angry with him, too.

             *Holly still wants Jane to tell her what to do.*
             *Jane ignores the request for guidance and*
             *uses a METACOMMUNICATION to focus on her*
             *feelings, while suggesting that Holly has some*
             *power in this relationship as well.*

Holly        I'm not a scary person.

Jane         Meaning Gary is?

             *Jane wants to know if there is an indication*
             *of domestic abuse.*

Holly        Well, he's six-one and pretty strong, so yeah, he can be.

             Time remaining
             25 minutes

Jane         Are you saying he might hit you?

             *Jane wants to find out if Holly is at risk*
             *because that would require a reassessment*
             *of the TREATMENT PLAN.*

| | |
|---|---|
| Holly | (Frowns slightly) No. He wouldn't. He never has. I just mean that he's scary when he's angry. I mean, usually he's cool, but when he loses his temper he just goes all Incredible Hulk. |
| Jane | The Incredible Hulk! You mean that character from the comics? |

*Jane dates herself here. This character is better known to Holly's generation for its appearance in contemporary movies and online than from the old comic strip from the 1960s or even the first TV series of the 1970s.*

| | |
|---|---|
| Holly | (Shakes her head) From the movie, yeah. |
| Jane | I see. So that makes you want to stay on his good side. Like walking on eggshells. Is that one of the reasons you developed the problem with your nerves? |

*Jane uses a cliché (walking on eggshells) as a RHETORICAL device to emphasize her point. She reverts, temporarily, to Holly's term, "nerves," to connect her question to Holly's original complaint.*

| | |
|---|---|
| Holly | I never thought of that. |
| Jane | You know what this reminds me of? The way you told me your father used to treat your mother. |

*This statement is an indirect INTERPRETATION.*

| | |
|---|---|
| Holly | Ha! You're right. And I'm just like my mother. |
| Jane | Out of the frying pan into the fire. The question is: are you going to wait 20 years before you stick up for yourself the way your mother finally did? |

*Another cliché but here the RHETORIC is not quite on point: it was her mother in the frying pan not her. Better not to overdo this TACTIC, lest it lose its effectiveness.*

Holly    I don't know if I'm even as strong as she is.

Jane    Yeah? Tell me about her. How is she a strong person?

*Jane wants to make use of the positive aspects of Holly's IDENTIFICATION with her mother.*

Holly    She just is.

Jane    Okay.

*Holly's inability to expand on her judgment about her mother may reflect the lag in abstracting ability, a normal part of adolescent development, rather than reluctance to elaborate on the topic. Jane avoids a critical comment but wants to continue the discussion.*

Holly    I mean, she raised me and my brothers. She stayed home and took care of us. She took care of the house and my father. Whatever. She waited, and then she did her own thing.

Jane    So it wasn't just your father making her stay home. She wanted to do it too.

*Holly makes an effort to elaborate but uses concrete examples rather than abstract observations, such as, for example: my mother is strong because she has an internal set of standards for herself and she sticks to them. Jane restates the description with a somewhat more abstract explanation.*

Holly        Yeah.

Jane         Well, stone the crows!

             *Another* RHETORICAL *attempt to strengthen
             her point, but this instance leads to a prob-
             lem instead.*

Holly        (Looks confused) What?

Jane         I just meant, "how about that!"

             *Jane makes an error in* DICTION *here.
             Instead of using the same type and level
             of language as Holly, she chooses a
             somewhat obscure expression completely
             outside of Holly's understanding. Like
             the "Incredible Hulk" reference earlier,
             Holly's unfamiliarity with the phrase cre-
             ates a distraction and undermines Jane's
             point.*

Holly        I thought you were thinking about Game of Thrones
             or something.

Jane         Sorry. I just got us off track. Go back to what you
             were saying about your mother.

             *Holly connects the phrase with a popular
             fantasy television drama which contains vari-
             ous references; for example, the Stone Crows
             tribe. Jane is unaware of the TV series, another
             example of unfamiliarity with Holly's frame of
             reference that can undermine the* THERAPEUTIC
             ALLIANCE. *She tries to recover from the disrup-
             tion her error caused.*

Holly        I'm not sure… what was I saying?

Jane        Your mother stayed home because she wanted to, not just because your father made her.

            *Holly does not return to the topic so Jane tries again.*

Holly       Oh, yeah. (Falls silent) Anyway, Gary's gonna come home tonight and then what?

Jane        You and Gary must have had fights before. What happened those other times?

            *The interruption caused by Jane's "stone the crows" comment has sealed off the exploration of parallels with Holly's parents. Jane gives up on the effort to talk about Holly's parents and tries to resume the earlier discussion.*

Holly       Mostly I just give in.

Jane        Is that what he'll expect this time too?

            *A FOUNDATION question.*

Holly       (Nodding) Probably.

Jane        You think you will?

            *This seemingly simple request for information contains the subtle implication that it would be a mistake if she does "give in."*

Holly       (Shakes her head and shrugs) Probably.

                                                    Time remaining
                                                    15 minutes

Jane        So you'll back down?

            *She REFRAMES Holly's "give in" using a term more relevant to the autonomy issue.*

Holly        I usually do.

Jane         I think what you're saying is that Gary has all the power and you have none.

> *Jane introduces a new idea, the balance of power in the relationship, as a FOUNDATION to later discussions about Holly's path to greater independence. She confronts Holly indirectly with the idea that she can use her power in the relationship, provided she asserts it.*

Holly        (Shrugs) Sounds about right.

Jane         And you're willing to live with that?

> *Jane is aware of feeling angry at this point. Her frustration derives from Holly's passivity and unwillingness to stand up for herself. Her reaction may stem from COUNTERTRANSFERENCE feelings: Jane's wish to see Holly as a different, more effective and more self-reliant person might result from Jane's inappropriate perception of Holly as a "little sister" or even a child. Another possibility is it could be an unconscious message Holly directs toward her, a PROVOKED EMOTION, a way for Holly to project her dependency feelings toward Jane. If Holly's responses have made Jane feel that way, it could be because Holly "intends" to generate a protective attitude in her by projecting a "poor helpless little me" image. Lacking evidence of COUNTERTRANSFERENCE, Jane will find it more useful to assume Holly "wants" her to feel frustrated and hopes Jane will respond with advice*

*and support. It occurs to her that Holly may act the same way with Gary, provoking him to tell her what to do.*

Holly        It's not really up to me.

Jane         Oh?

             *With this simple expression, Jane avoids ask-ing "why" Holly feels that way, since "why" questions tend to come across as criticism.*

Holly        No, I'm a go-along-to-get-along type of person.

Jane         And you're happy with that?

             *Holly puts into words a part of her identity that underpins her problems with overde-pendence. Jane's FOUNDATIONAL question contains the idea that Holly could change the dynamic if she wanted to.*

Holly        Not really, but that's just how I am.

Jane         (Shaking her head) Well, here's a news flash:you don't have to be that kind of person.

             *Holly further reveals that this trait is EGO SYNTONIC. Before she can modify it, she must first see it as undesirable (EGO DYSTONIC). Jane makes overt the idea: Holly has power in the relationship but she has to recognize and employ it.*

Holly        I don't?

Jane         No.

Holly     And how am I supposed to change?

Jane      Well, first you have to want to.

> *Again, Holly looks for advice, but at least she accepts the idea that a change might be needed. Jane declines to give advice and challenges Holly to accept the responsibility for change.*

Holly     Yeah, but what if I change and then my marriage falls apart? I don't want that.

Time remaining
5 minutes

Jane      Why should it?

> *The NEGATIVE OVERGENERALIZATION reemerges.*

> *Although this is a "why" question, the query is about an abstraction, the marriage, and is not a question about personal behavior, so the "why" is less judgmental.*

Holly     Well, because if I change too much, I won't be the girl he married.

Jane      So then he won't love you anymore?

> *If Jane utilized a COGNITIVE-BEHAVIORAL approach here, she might invite Holly to explore the proposition: I must put my needs second to others or they will abandon me.*

Holly     Yeah.

Jane      I see. But couldn't it work the other way, too? Maybe he'd prefer somebody with backbone, somebody who stands up for herself, somebody who—

Holly        (Forcefully) You're crazy. Obviously, you don't
             know Gary!

Jane         No, that's true. Everything I know about Gary is
             based on what you tell me. That's your idea of Gary.
             Maybe he's not exactly the person you think he is.

             *When Holly interrupts Jane, "the authority,"
             and disagrees with her she shows a spark of
             backbone. A welcome sign. Making the point
             that Holly's version of Gary may be dis-
             torted LAYS A FOUNDATION for a later discus-
             sion of this possibility in more depth.*

Holly        After five years I think I know him pretty well.

Jane         Here's something to think about: the way Gary treats
             you may be based on how you act toward him. If you
             go all weak and helpless, and send him the message
             that you're just a helpless child who needs him to take
             care of her, if you send him the message that you need
             somebody to tell you what to do, then that makes
             Gary be the grown-up. He has to be in charge because
             you aren't. He has to make the decisions and decide
             what's best, because you don't give him any choice.

             *One effect of Jane's contention that Holly
             has provoked Gary to be domineering is to
             raise the idea that, since Holly is responsible
             (at least in part) for his behavior, she has
             the power to change the relationship. In this
             explanation she adopts a TRANSACTIONAL
             THERAPY model of behavior.*

Holly        No, that's not right. Look what happened when I
             talked about getting a job. He didn't appreciate me
             doing that.

Jane            When people are used to acting one way, they don't change right away when the other person tries to change.

> *Jane counters with a NORMATIVE statement. She implies that Holly may alter the balance of power if she persists.*

Holly           (Discouraged) I don't know.

Jane            Our time is up for today and we have to stop.

Holly           Okay. (She sits for a moment, evidently thinking about what Jane has told her, then she nods, gets up and turns toward the door) See you next week.

### Discussion

One of the therapy goals, and the one Holly is most interested in, is to minimize the anxiety symptoms that were her reason for seeking help from the clinic, and yet, in both the previous session and this one, her references to her anxiety have almost disappeared without any specific therapeutic work.

One possible reason for this change: the anxiety symptom, while real, was an "admission ticket," a legitimate reason for Holly to seek help for the more nebulous and abstract problems of her new marriage and her isolation from friends and family. Since she is now in treatment and getting help, she no longer needs to talk about this symptom, at least for that reason. The presenting complaint often serves this purpose and its disappearance or rapid resolution is a common occurrence in psychotherapy practice. Without a formulation and a treatment plan that addresses the underlying problems, resolution of the presenting symptom might lead to the conclusion that the client is now okay. Termination would be premature, leaving the important issues unaddressed.

Another possibility: Holly's acceptance for therapy and the initial conditions of her treatment (the promise of expert help, of regular appointments, and of a therapeutic structure) promoted a placebo effect. This kind of improvement, in the absence of more focused efforts to ameliorate the problem, may prove only temporary or it may turn out to be the foundation of more lasting progress.

The therapeutic alliance may have provided symbolic relief if Holly experienced the therapy relationship as nurturing, protective and safe, conditions whose absence fueled her anxiety symptoms before treatment. These expectations could later lead to a transference problem if Holly sees Jane as a "mother figure," but, in fact, nurturance, protection and safety are authentic features of therapy.[5] As such, they are not distortions but valuable aspects of the alliance.

The work Jane and Holly did in the previous session seems to be paying off in Holly's early indications that she is willing to be more independent. The "big fight" that Holly was so anxious to tell Jane about was ostensibly set off by the question of whether Holly should get a job. A job would mean a challenge to Gary's authority by asserting her own. The threat to earn money herself would undermine Gary's position as "the breadwinner" and the person with ultimate control over spending. Holly would leave the safety of the home and confront the uncertainties of life in the outside adult world. Holly has accepted that Jane does not give advice and does not shrink from considering on her own what she might do. That indicates real progress.

Although the topic of child-bearing did not arise in this session, Holly's interest in work outside the home has a bearing on the disagreement with Gary over children. Gary has been pushing to start a family immediately. Holly wants to delay, but she had used her problem with "nerves" as a reason. If she goes out to work, she would delay pregnancy, not because she was "sick," a position of weakness, but because she chooses to wait, a position of strength.

In the argument with Gary, Holly tried to shift onto Jane the responsibility for the idea of waiting and, at least in this session, Jane did not confront her about it, even though her deception deflected some of Gary's anger away from Holly and toward Jane. Perhaps Jane felt that the benefit of standing up to Gary outweighed the complications arising from shifting the responsibility to her, and that, later, when she felt stronger and more confident, Holly could take full responsibility for her decision. Holly was not wrong in her conclusion that Jane wanted her to do it, even though job-hunting was not mentioned as part of the treatment plan, because of Jane's responses during the prior session; for instance, how strongly Jane challenged Holly's statement, "if Gary'd let me." Jane shifted from a psychodynamic stance to a cognitive-behavioral one when she recognized the impact of Holly's negative overgeneralization ("Unless I do everything he says, Gary will abandon me") on her marital relationship.

Jane began a major intervention when she attempted to redefine the marital relationship as one in which Holly invites and provokes Gary's domineering behavior by her passivity and projected helplessness. If Gary is an unregenerate bully and Holly is simply a passive, helpless victim, the therapy will have no path to help Holly develop as an adult and no alternative for her but to leave the marriage and move on. But if Holly can accept the idea that she is, at least in part, the cause of Gary's attitude toward her, then, by changing the way she relates to him, she can change his behavior toward her. In other words, in this transactional model, if Holly is the cause of the imbalance, then she is in a position to improve it.

When Jane became aware, about two-thirds of the way through the session, that she felt angry at Holly's willingness to accept her second-class status in the marriage, she was able to recognize a behavioral tactic that Holly uses to generate sympathy and caretaking from others, presumably her parents and possibly her friends as well as Gary. In other words, Holly presents herself as needy and helpless in order to get others to take responsibility for her. Jane can use this transactional hypothesis for further exploration and, if confirmed, as a focus of her therapeutic efforts.

The question of Jane's influence on what Holly may choose to do, not only about working outside the home, but about the marriage in general, raises the possibility that Jane is under the influence of countertransference distortions. If Jane finds herself with a covert agenda—for example, that Holly would be better off without Gary; in other words, divorced—that recognition should serve as a warning that her own feelings have intruded where they do not belong. Divorce rates for teenage marriages are the highest of any age group (Kiernan, 1986) but statistics do not apply to the individual, and Holly's marriage may prove durable and rewarding. Jane, an educated, independent woman, might resent Gary's attempt to terminate Holly's therapy and harbor a poor opinion of him, concluding (with no evidence) that he is a lower-class boor oppressing his wife.

Jane should not take sides. She must avoid judgment about Gary and about the marriage because she has only Holly's version of events and only her side of any argument. Even if Holly does not consciously distort the facts in an attempt to manipulate Jane, her version of events may differ significantly from what really happened and, in any case, is likely to contrast with Gary's version. Jane only "knows" Gary through Holly's reports, and he may be a somewhat different person from how his wife portrays him.

Jane should not be, and indeed cannot be, a parent or an advocate for what she might believe would be best for Holly. Not only would such a stance ignore Holly's right to make her own decisions, but, lacking both a first-hand knowledge of Holly's situation and god-like omniscience, Jane could easily get it wrong. Her bias would distort her role as a therapist and could do real harm to Holly.

## Notes

1 The use of "because" in this formulation demonstrates how cause-and-effect connections generate treatment plans.
2 See the chapter "General Principles of Psychotherapy."
3 A simple schema for psychodynamic psychotherapy work is: identification, clarification, confrontation, interpretation.
4 An inaccurate interpretation has the opposite effect, resulting in an easy acceptance and creating feelings of relief, because the patient recognizes that it will not disturb his or her psychic equilibrium.
5 The chapter "General Principles of Psychotherapy" reviews Frank's ideas about "healing and persuasion" that underlie those three characteristics of the therapeutic relationship.

## Reference

Kiernan, K. E. (1986). Teenage marriage and marital breakdown: A longitudinal study. *Population Studies*, 40(1), 35–54.

# George

## An Unsettled Graduate Student

## Referral

George was initially seen at the university Student Health Service. His visit was in response to his girlfriend's concern that he was "depressed and having suicidal thoughts." Because of the perceived risk he was seen immediately by the on-call clinician. After his intake interview he was referred to Jane with the following brief report:

This 27 year old unmarried male graduate student was seen on an urgent visit because of depression with suicidal ideation. He is enrolled in the Master of Arts in Religion program at the Divinity School. He will receive his degree in May. Over the past two months he has been mildly depressed and revealed to his girlfriend that he was having thoughts of "ending it all." Apparently he has been struggling with classes and burdened by his teaching assistant duties. He feels isolated and alone. His postgraduate goals are vague. He thinks he might go into management at a non-profit organization or look for a job with an overseas non-government association. His relationship with his girlfriend, Alice, also a student at the Divinity School, has been strained because she does not want to begin a sexual relationship until she is married.

In the interview he was a pleasant, well-spoken man who appeared somewhat shy and uncomfortable. He denied past history of depression, suicidal behavior, psychosis or hospitalization. He has no suicide plan. His depressed mood seemed to grow out of a general dissatisfaction and unhappiness with his

DOI: 10.4324/9781003353003-5

current life circumstances. Beck Depression Inventory was in the low range at 15.

Impression: Depression, mild, single episode (F32.0)
Plan: Hospitalization deferred
Refer for individual psychotherapy

Jane picked up his referral and saw him at the Student Health Clinic. Her assessment concurred with the referral that risk of self-harm was low. At their first meeting she gathered some additional background.

## History

George is the younger of two brothers from an intact, professional family. His father is an attorney working in intellectual property law. His mother is in cancer research at the medical school. (Jane does not know her.) He had an apparently unremarkable childhood, but one that included regular Church attendance and devout observance at home. George had good grades throughout school and graduated college with a cum laude BA degree. Never a good athlete, he considered himself a "nerd" and was active in computer-oriented activities and chess club as after-school activities. He developed superficial relationships through these interests but had no close friendships and did not date until college. After college he was uncertain what to do next and spent the following three years working in a supermarket as an assistant manager. His parents encouraged him to get a graduate degree and he went along with the idea but without much enthusiasm. He chose the Divinity School at the urging of his parents, but he does not feel he fits in there and says he is "just marking time." He met Alice, his current girlfriend, in a Divinity School class and they have been dating casually for three months. Alice is "a good Christian" who wants to maintain her virginity until sanctified by marriage. George is also sexually inexperienced.

## Formulation

Jane's hypothesis is that George shows evidence of identity diffusion, a condition sometimes associated with borderline personality disorder, although George shows no evidence (at this early stage) of the latter diagnosis. Nevertheless, his current challenges seem to lie in the areas of resolving conflicts between his parents' religious lifestyle and his more secular inclinations, between his academic pursuits and his interest in a management career, and between his self-sufficient social life and the pull of more gregarious social and sexual activities. While it is not unusual for young adults to work out their identity issues over a period of years (Fadjukoff et al., 2016), George seems to have stalled in the face of these challenges and remains discouraged and confused about his path forward.

(Formulation Category: Developmental)

## Treatment Plan

Jane settled on resolving his indecision as the *aim* of her work with George. She does not select identity consolidation itself as the desired outcome because that process may take years and George plans to leave the university and the area in a few months. Treatment *goals* will include elucidation of the factors impeding his growth, broadening his social network, especially with regard to more support, and helping him resolve his ambivalence toward Alice and females in general. As to *strategy*, she intends to take an exploratory path using psychodynamic principles. She discusses these ideas with George and he agrees, somewhat half-heartedly, but Jane feels they have enough of a treatment contract to begin work together.

## Early Progress

During the first four sessions, Jane pursues her treatment objectives through additional history about George's family and his experiences with the family's religious activities. They have discussed his difficulties with the social environment from grade school through college. George has talked about his current relationship with Alice. Jane has the impression that George is simply going through the motions and that he has not absorbed much of the progress she hoped they would see.

Of concern, however, Jane has noticed that George tends to stare at her body, especially her breasts and legs, even though she dresses conservatively in styles that do not include low necklines or raised hems; in fact, she usually wears a jacket over a high-necked blouse and a mid-calf length skirt or slacks. Because George's staring behavior does not so far seem to be a therapy problem she has not yet addressed it.

## SESSION FIVE

Unlike his presentation in earlier sessions, when he has been relaxed and acting a little bored, today George appears agitated. He is dressed casually—if not sloppily—in a loose sweatshirt stamped with the school's logo and a wrinkled pair of loose cotton pants. He paces the room before taking his chair and does not make eye contact with Jane. When seated he leans forward, clasping his hands in his lap and staring out the window.

Time remaining
45 minutes

Jane    You seem to have a lot on your mind today. What's going on?

*George conveys his inner turmoil by how he dresses and moves, rather than in words. Jane acknowledges his non-verbal distress with a* METACOMMUNICATION *and asks him to put it into words. Given his evident distress she discards her own plan for the session in order to deal with whatever upset George is going through.*

George    (Looks at her) Are you a Christian?

Jane    Is that important?

*An unexpected beginning. George appears to want to "prequalify" her before*

*he reveals more. She avoids a "why"*
*question ("Why do you ask?") and uses a*
*METACOMMUNICATION to explore the source*
*of his question.*

George   I just need to know how you're going to react to something I want to discuss with you.

Jane   And whether I'm a Christian would make a difference?

> *Jane isn't sure whether his question is a*
> *BOUNDARY VIOLATION (an inappropriate*
> *inquiry into her personal history) or a*
> *renegotiation of the THERAPEUTIC CONTRACT.*
> *Some devout patients feel they need a therapist*
> *of the same religion to be fully understood.*

George   Christianity is all about forgiveness. I guess that's what I'm asking about.

Jane   Whether I would forgive you? Do you think that's my role?

> *Her question implies that their therapeutic*
> *contract is **not** one of penitent–confessor.*

George   (Shakes his head in frustration) Something upsetting happened and I don't know how you'd take it.

Jane   Why don't you just tell me about it and we'll go from there.

> *She might have used a METACOMMUNICATION,*
> *such as "What do you think my reaction will*
> *be?" but she chooses a more direct inquiry*
> *so that they can get right to whatever it is he*
> *is hesitant to reveal.*

George          I guess so. (He pauses, apparently struggling for words) Well, okay... I was almost arrested last night...

Jane            (When he doesn't go on) For what?

                *Again, she opts for a direct inquiry, given the level of emotional upset he is experiencing.*

George          (Grimaces) This is hard... Okay, here's what happened. I live in an apartment building where you can go up to the roof. It's a flat roof with a waist-high wall around the edge, so it's like a... a roof picnic area or something. So I go up there at night if I'm feeling upset or whatever. Or sometimes just to get some fresh air. So I was up there last night and walking back and forth and the people in the top floor apartment must have heard me walking around and they called the police. So all of a sudden these two cops come through the door with their guns out and put their flashlights on me. And I'm like, hey, what's going on. (He stops and stares at his hands in his lap) So, finally, I tell them I live in the building and they march me down to my apartment and they see I have a key and I show them my student ID and so finally they leave.

Jane            Is there more to it? Because I don't see where you'd need forgiveness for that. It sounds like it was just a misunderstanding.

                *He seems to be CATASTROPHIZING a merely unpleasant event. Jane suspects there is more to it.*

George          Yeah, you're right. There's more. That's the hard part.

Jane            Can you tell me that part?

*She continues to encourage him directly since she needs the full history behind his description of a somewhat awkward but otherwise benign-sounding event.*

George   So, when I go up there... (his face blushes a deep pink and then he speaks in a rush) When-I-go-up-there-I-look-into-windows. At the other buildings. I'm looking to see women undress or whatever. I'm being a... Peeping Tom.

Jane   And that's the part you feel guilty about? That's why you need forgiveness?

*She accepts the strength of his feelings by putting them into words for him.*

George   Can you imagine what would happen if they caught me doing that? I'd be disgraced. I'd be kicked out of my program. My life would be over. Oh, God! (He begins to sob)

Jane   That does sound serious.

*She acknowledges the magnitude of the problem, hoping this will help him discuss it more openly. Jane also wonders whether this new information creates a duty to warn.[1] She will listen for any hint that George has targeted a specific person.*

George   (Wipes his face with his hands) I'm all fucked up.

Jane   But from what you told me, the police were satisfied that you weren't a threat and they didn't arrest you for peeping.

*On the face of it, this encounter with the police ended without consequence. Since*

> *it was not the CATASTROPHE he imagines,*
> *Jane suggests indirectly that his reaction is*
> *disproportionate in the hopes that he will*
> *reveal more about his fears.*

George   Yeah, not this time, but what if it happens again?

Jane   Do you still plan to go up to the roof?

> *Taking a cognitive-behavioral approach,*
> *she challenges what appears to be his*
> *OVERGENERALIZATION to the event.*

George   (Shakes his head) I wouldn't take the chance.

Jane   Then, what's the problem?

> *Jane strongly suspects that the problem is*
> *his career as a Peeping Tom, since this kind*
> *of impulse-driven behavior is usually long-*
> *standing and pervasive. She wants him to*
> *confront the issue himself.*

George   The problem is I don't know if I can stop. If I see an opportunity I just, I just do it, you know. It's like a compulsion. I don't know if I can stop myself.

Jane   Ah, a compulsion. I see what you mean. Have you ever been arrested? Any other run-ins with the police?

> *First, as a matter of DICTION, Jane notes*
> *his use of "compulsion" to describe his*
> *problem. She will use that word, his word, in*
> *future discussions. By using his own term for*
> *his voyeurism, she hopes to better connect*
> *with him about his problem. Second, if he*
> *already has a criminal record, his prognosis*
> *would be less promising. She wonders if*
> *she might still be able to work with him,*

*although the threat of a subsequent arrest might be even more motivating.*

George   No. Never. This thing last night was the first time I had the police come after me.

Jane   That's helpful to know.

*She reinforces his apparent willingness to talk freely about his behavior, recognizing that, if she agrees to treat him, she will need an uncensored history in order to create a new treatment plan.*

Time remaining
35 minutes

George   Well, I need to keep it that way. (Shivers) So how do we do this? Can you help me?

Jane   We can certainly try. Let's start with what happens here in the office. I've noticed from time to time you tend to stare at me. Is that the same thing? A compulsion?

*The real question is not what Jane can do for him, but rather what he can do for himself. She lets that misperception slide for the moment since she is still collecting data. Now that he admits the extent of the problem, she brings it into the therapy by noting his behavior toward her, a tactic not without risk: can she be both his therapist and the object of his compulsion? If she ignores his staring at her, making her a sexual object, would that undermine her therapeutic role? Should she incorporate this behavior in the new treatment plan? Should she recommend a male therapist? She feels uncertain about the therapeutic path she has started down.*

George        (Blushes) I know, I know. I shouldn't be doing that.

Jane          So that's something about yourself you want to change?

*This new information requires a new FORMULATION (a change from the "Developmental" category to "Transactional") and thus a renegotiation of the TREATMENT CONTRACT. One hopeful indication is that his behavior appears EGO DYSTONIC. He blushes with shame each time he admits a new instance. His distress is not solely due to his fear of arrest and social disgrace but also seems to be a part of himself that he dislikes. At least, Jane hopes that's what his blushing indicates.*

George        Do you think I can?

Jane          Sexual compulsions are difficult to treat. It's not an area where I've had much experience. Would you rather I refer you to someone more knowledgeable about helping with this kind of problem?

*The first step in the renegotiation is to recognize that she cannot provide her usual level of expertise, with the implication that she might not be able to help him with what she correctly identifies as a difficult type of behavior for him to change.*

George        Somebody else? (Shakes his head) No, I'd rather not. I feel comfortable talking to you. I don't want to have to go through this with somebody new.

Jane          Even if you didn't get as good a result from the ther-
              apy as you hoped?

              *She wants to give him every chance to accept
              a referral. She realizes she could decline to
              continue with his treatment, but she thinks he
              might not contact anyone else on her referral
              list or would quickly drop out and end up with
              no therapy at all. In addition, she believes from
              the prior sessions that they have a connection,
              a good* THERAPEUTIC ALLIANCE *(which his
              last statement seems to confirm), and that she
              could work with him. Finally, she will note in
              his chart that she suggested a referral and he
              declined. If this effort results in a malpractice
              suit,* [2] *she will have this record for her defense.*

George        (Stubbornly) I don't want to go to somebody else.

Jane          How about if we could find a twelve-step program for
              you?

              *She's not aware of any specific peer group
              resources although she thinks one might be
              helpful, even if it is an adjunct to the therapy
              with her.*

George        (Frowns) You mean like AA? I don't think I could do
              that. Get up in front of people and talk about it? No way.

Jane          Okay. Well, let's keep that in our back pocket and see
              how far we get in here.

              *She realizes he is not open to any other
              avenues of treatment so she decides to continue
              with him for his "compulsion" but now has to
              determine how they will work on it.*

George    So how do we do this?

Jane    Well, one thing to think about is whether medication could help. Sometimes antidepressants can be useful.

> *Jane continues to renegotiate, offering a new strategy. Some antidepressants have the side effect of dampening the patient's libido, a change that might reduce the inner voyeuristic pressure.*

George    I don't want to take any pills. Back when I was in high school, my regular doctor gave me some kind of antidepressant. It made me feel weird. Fuzzy and kind of out of it. I threw them away.

Jane    What was going on then, that he thought you needed medication?

> *This is more new information. She pauses the negotiation to find out more about it. She avoids a why question (Why did you need an antidepressant back then?) that might imply disapproval.*

George    It was my parents' idea. They thought I was moping around too much. Which I was. I didn't have friends in high school. I spent a lot of time in my room. I was into online games and stuff like that.

Jane    Were you depressed? Did you have suicidal thoughts? It sounds more like you were unhappy.

> *If it now turns out he really has a history of depression, often a recurring illness, she wants to know about it. If so, she needs to reassess suicide risk.*

George      Suicidal thoughts? No way. I just was happier on my own. I wasn't like the other kids. I never felt I belonged.

Jane      Okay, well let's get back to the question of how we're going to proceed. You don't want to see someone else and you don't want to take medication. That limits what we can do together.

> *It sounds like he was inappropriately treated by his doctor. Jane could continue to pursue this information but the more important objective right now is the new treatment plan.*

George      What about just regular therapy?

Jane      Okay. The therapy that might work the best is called cognitive-behavioral. It means primarily two things. First, we'd look at how your thoughts about this area of your life affect your sexual behavior. And second, we'd look for how you can change your behavior in order to minimize the pressure you feel to do your peeping.

> *Jane outlines a specific STRATEGY because she wants him to be fully aware of what they will do to work on his problem. She uses the term "peeping" instead of "voyeurism" to match his DICTION.*

George      Yeah, I've heard about that. CBT, right?

Jane      Right. We'd look for specific things you could do to modify this problem.

> *So the new strategy would be a directive approach. Jane wants to nail down their agreement about how to proceed.*

George       And you think that will work?

Jane         We'll have to see.

>            *Actually, she is skeptical, given how hard it is*
>            *to modify impulse control problems. Although*
>            *she wants to maximize whatever* PLACEBO
>            EFFECT *results from this new direction, she*
>            *doesn't want to "guarantee" a result.*

George       (He has a determined expression) Okay.

Jane         So let's begin with something simple and direct. We
             talked about the way you stare at my chest or at other
             parts of me. That's a good example of your inner
             pressure in this area, your compulsion, and it's right
             here in the office where we can see how successful
             you can be with our treatment program. So, what I
             want you to do is be aware of when you feel inclined
             to stare and consciously block yourself from doing it.
             At the same time, we need to know that you're fight-
             ing the impulse, so signal me by raising one finger.

>            *Jane initiates an exposure and response*
>            *prevention exercise to see directly how*
>            *successful that* TACTIC *might be. Also, she*
>            *doesn't like his staring and wants it to stop.*
>            *Adding the instruction to raise his finger to*
>            *signal his awareness of his impulse not only*
>            *allows her to track his behavioral impulse but*
>            *also adds a negative reinforcement; namely,*
>            *that he must physically show (to his apparent*
>            *shame) that he has had an unacceptable*
>            *impulse. This part of the exercise is an*
>            *example of* PARADOXICAL INTENTION.

George       (Looking out the window) What are you going to do
             if it happens?

Time remaining
25 minutes

Jane          Are you worried that I'll criticize you?

*She responds with a METACOMMUNICATION
in the form of a question. Once he knows
she is aware of his staring behavior, Jane
expects that he will try to fight it out of fear
of criticism or shaming. She wants him to
take on the exercise as the beginning effort
to control his voyeuristic impulses and block
them because he finds them unacceptable,
modifying his inner "conscience" control,
rather than because of external risk. As a
test, if he can control himself in front of her
she will be more confident he can do so in
other circumstances.*

George        Well, yeah. You don't want me to do it, right? You're
              telling me to stop.

Jane          Not exactly. If you relied on me to tell you to stop,
              well… two things. One, I won't be with you when you
              have this impulse and you're not in my office, so that
              wouldn't work, and, two, if you only stopped because
              I said so, you'd never develop the self-control you'll
              need to stop yourself from doing it. The idea is for you
              to develop more control over this behavior and here's
              a simple drill that can help you make a start on that.

*She hopes to educate him with this statement.
She tries to spell it out for him without
acknowledging that, yes, she doesn't like it, but
the more important reason is to get him started
on the new STRATEGY. She feels that sharing
her personal dislike of his staring at her body
would only weaken the alliance and undermine*

> *the potential progress it offers him. Jane is*
> *flirting here with a BOUNDARY VIOLATION*
> *(seeing her as a sexual object) that is the*
> *background of this part of their relationship, by*
> *making herself part of the exercise.*

George        Okay. I'll give it a shot.

Jane          Let's try it out right now. Look at me and tell me
              what goes through your mind and then exert your
              control over it.

> *She asks him to demonstrate his compliance*
> *with the proposed TACTIC and also to make*
> *his behavior part of the process of the*
> *therapy.*

George        (Looks at her chest) I feel stupid doing this like
              that.

Jane          Besides that. What is your thought?

> *She wants to be sure he recognizes the*
> *cognitive component of his attraction.*

George        (Reluctantly) I'm wondering what they look like. (He
              turns his head and looks at the window) Now I'm not
              looking.

Jane          You don't have to say it in words. Raise your finger
              when you feel you have it under control.

> *His willingness to signal when he is exerting*
> *control is an important component of the*
> *exercise.*

George        (Raises his finger, still looking away)

| Jane | Okay, so that's how it works. (She waits until he looks back at her and lowers his finger) Now I'd like to learn more about the background of this problem. Like, when did it start? In what circumstances are you feeling most tempted by it? Whether you ever got into trouble because of it. |
|---|---|

*She wants to gather a history of this specific problem in order to have the material from which to build a behavior modification program.*

| George | (Sits back in his chair) It started when I was a teenager. This girl lived in the house next door to me. Her room faced my house and I could see into her windows, especially at night when the lights were on. Sometimes she left the curtains open or they weren't all the way closed and I could see into her bedroom. So I got in the habit of watching for those chances. I'd be standing by my window waiting for a chance to see something. Most of the time I wouldn't see anything but every once in a while I'd get a glimpse. |
|---|---|

| Jane | It sounds like that took up a lot of your time— |
|---|---|

| George | (Interjects) Hours! I wasted hours every time but I couldn't stop myself. |
|---|---|

| Jane | Yes, you could have been doing other things. Did your homework suffer? Did you see less of your family? |
|---|---|

*Jane wants to highlight the cost of this behavior as an indication of the possible reward of freeing himself from this activity.*

| George | (Ruefully) That's all true. |
|---|---|

Jane — How old was this girl?

> *She wants to check whether his voyeurism has an underlying pedophilia.*

George — She was around my age. She was in the class behind me.

Jane — Okay. So what happened next?

> *She asks for additional history of peeping, looking for ANTECEDENTS and triggers for the behavior. A teenage boy spying on the girl next door isn't yet full-blown voyeurism.*

George — Nothing happened. I went away to school. I didn't see that girl anymore.

Jane — I meant, what happened after that. When does your compulsion crop up? What's the next time you remember?

> *Jane wonders if he "misunderstood" her question out of a reluctance to reveal more or if he really didn't understand her question. So far, he's been forthcoming but she suspects more problematic voyeuristic episodes have occurred that may be harder for him to talk about.*

George — I never snuck around people's houses looking into windows or anything like that. (He blinks rapidly, then looks over at the window and raises his finger)

Jane — Looks like you caught yourself and then controlled it. I didn't even see you staring this time.

> *She acknowledges his successful response as a reinforcement.*

George       I was about to look and then I didn't.

Jane       That's a success. And that's how we'll work on this problem.

> *She continues to reinforce his use of the exercise. She then* RENAMES *his behavior as a "problem." It might be better to continue calling it "peeping" or even introduce the term "voyeurism" as a way to support his motivation to change. Using a shadow word like "compulsion" is a way to avoid fully confronting the behavior. She also notes that his "compliance" with the exercise allowed him to avoid telling her about other voyeuristic events, as she had asked about.*

George       (Shrugs and nods) Yeah, it's not so hard to do it in here. What about when I'm on my own?

Time remaining
15 minutes

Jane       That remains to be seen, doesn't it? Remember, you're not going up to the roof anymore. What other kinds of situations are tempting you now?

> *Jane asks again about other episodes, this time in the form of temptations rather than actual events. She wants to catalog his behavior outside the office in order to design a more specific program of control for him.*

George       Nothing now. Going up to the roof was the only thing I was doing.

Jane       I see. Well, one thing we haven't talked about is how all this affects your relationship with Alice.

Does she know about it? Do you try to look at her that way?

> *Jane wonders if he is being truthful about no other voyeuristic activities. His initial strong motivation to work with her on his problem seems to be fading as they get into difficult areas of his history. Rather than confronting him now, she asks about his current girlfriend as a way to begin to explore his other sexual behaviors. Is the voyeurism fueled by his lack of other outlets? What are the ANTECEDENTS of that behavior?*

George   I told you, Alice is... She's not into sex outside of marriage. Sure, I'd like to see her naked, but that's not where it's going.

Jane   So, you're okay with that?

> *She wonders if his frustration with Alice adds to the pressure to peep at other women.*

George   Not really, but I like her. And, actually, I'd be kind of afraid to get into that with her. I... I don't have much experience in that area.

Jane   Would you say that Alice is kind of a safe relationship for you?

> *This question is actually an INTERPRETATION. How helpful this line of inquiry would be to the therapy she is trying to design is questionable.*

George   Safe? I don't know what you mean by that.

| Jane | I mean, Alice doesn't require you to manage a sexual relationship, but at the same time, lack of sex with Alice might make you feel you need to look at other women more. |
|---|---|

*Jane tries to recover by suggesting that her question was a FOUNDATION: does his lack of sex with Alice fuel the pressure he feels to peep?*

| George | I see. (Thinks) I don't know. I'd have to think about that. |
|---|---|

| Jane | Another question. Do you watch any pornography? |
|---|---|

*She abandons this line of inquiry as unproductive. Her question about pornography LAYS A FOUNDATION for an idea she has about another intervention.*

| George | Pornography? I wouldn't know how to do that. |
|---|---|

| Jane | It's online. I believe it's one of the most common things people do with their smart phones and tablets. |
|---|---|

*Jane wonders if, knowing his history with computers, he is lying. A voyeur who claims not even to know about pornography seems unlikely. She chooses not to confront him, given the risk to the THERAPEUTIC ALLIANCE. Instead, she offers an informational and normalizing statement.*

| George | I didn't know that. |
|---|---|

| Jane | Okay, well, we're getting near the end of our time today. I'd like you to work on a couple of things before our next session. |
|---|---|

*She wants him to use the time between*
*sessions to carry out the TACTICS they*
*develop in their discussions in the office.*

George        (Frowns) Like homework?

Jane          Yes, exactly. Like homework. The first thing I'd like
              you to do is to write down a detailed history of your
              peeping experiences. Preferably in chronological
              order, maybe starting with the girl next door that you
              told me about earlier and continuing right up to the
              present, your going up to your roof to look in win-
              dows. Can you do that?

                         *She acknowledges that it's "homework," a*
                         *name that is consistent with the directive*
                         *approach she has decided to use. He has*
                         *been unwilling to tell her about past episodes*
                         *and writing them down may be easier than*
                         *saying them out loud. Asking for a written*
                         *history will also save time in the session and*
                         *provide the data for further TACTICS. It may*
                         *prove therapeutic in that it requires him to*
                         *reveal and confront his history.*

George        Why would you need me to do that?

                                                    Time remaining
                                                    5 minutes

Jane          Having that information will help us figure out what
              you can do to control it. Like what we did earlier
              with you looking at me and raising your finger when
              you were able to stop it. If we can figure the kinds of
              things that trigger you to start peeping we can look
              for ways to head it off before it becomes a risky situ-
              ation where you might get caught.

*She provides some educational basis for
the assignment to help motivate him to
complete the task. She ignores his reluctance
to write it down. A* METACOMMUNICATION
*such as "do you have any worries about this
assignment?" would have helped uncover
any resistance to this important exercise.*

George     Okay. Should I email it to you?

Jane       (Shakes her head) No. Write it down with pen and
           paper. We don't want this information to have any
           chance to be seen by anyone else. Not on your com-
           puter. Not in cyberspace.

           *Jane is surprised he doesn't recognize this
           risk. He seems unusually naïve for a graduate
           student. She wonders how that might play into
           his problems with sex and relationships, but
           that isn't the focus of their work at this point.*

George     Oh, right. I didn't think of that.

Jane       So, that's the first thing. The other homework assign-
           ment is more in the category of an exercise. I want
           you to find some online pornography and explore
           what kinds of things you like to watch on it.

           *She wants to see if an alternative sexual outlet
           lessens the compulsion to peep and diverts him
           from his high risk behavior. Weakening the
           impulse is not as good as controlling it, but
           because of his legal jeopardy if he continues
           to act on it, anything that reduces his inner
           pressure will be helpful.*

George     Really? That's not illegal, is it?

| Jane | Yes, really. And no, it's not illegal. The idea with that is to have you express your sexual interest in a safe, private environment. You can't be arrested for watching it. At least, if you don't include any child pornography. That **would** be illegal and very risky, but from what you've said you don't have any interest in children. So, stick to adults and let's see if that takes some of the pressure off. |
| | *Again, she gives an educational rationale and then, given how naïve he seems, warns him about the legal limits involved.* |

| George | (Looks conflicted, but then nods his head) Okay, I got it. |

| Jane | Good. Well, our time is up for today and we have to stop. |

Jane has not explored his obvious RESISTANCE to her plan and time has run out.


### *Discussion*

A rather straightforward course of therapy, one focused on George's school and interpersonal problems, is suddenly upended by his revelation of a longstanding pervasive sexual disorder with potentially devastating consequences. Voyeurism is a crime. Whether it is a misdemeanor or a felony depends on the jurisdiction and the accompanying circumstances. As George realizes, an arrest would have dire consequences for his educational plans, his acceptance within his society, and could even include a possible prison sentence and placement on the Sexual Offenders List. The stakes are high for treatment to succeed.

The diagnosis on record, from the original referral note after George was seen for an urgent visit, is "mild depression." Based on the new information, the correct diagnosis should be Voyeuristic Disorder (F65.3). Jane does not want to place such a pejorative term in the school's official records. Although medical records are confidential and protected under the HIPPA[3] laws, these protections are not absolute and subject to gossip by health personnel, theft by computer hacking and legal inquiry. Jane decides to leave the existing diagnosis in place and not subject George to any additional risk.

Jane must also consider her duty to warn. In this interview, George has not identified a specific person that he "peeps" at. The duty to warn does not include past acts nor does it cover general behavior not directed at an individual. Since no one has been identified as at risk, Jane is not required to warn anyone. She failed to educate George on this duty, which she should do at their next meeting. If he is forewarned about the risk it may strengthen his control over this behavior, although it could also make him even more reluctant to tell her of any current activities.

Another problem is Jane's lack of prior training or experience with treating voyeurism. The easier choice would be to refer George to a more experienced therapist or a specific treatment program. Jane does not know where either of these resources could be found, but hopes she could locate one or more by research and networking. For example, she could post a message on the medical school email list asking for the information.

The problems George has created for Jane originate from his lack of candor. To put it bluntly, he lied by omission when he did not mention his voyeurism. He may have lied again when he claimed to know nothing about online pornography. Jane must now worry about possible other lies in what George has told her. Discovery of the lies has weakened the therapeutic alliance.

Because of the new history, Jane must now change her formulation. Serious interpersonal difficulties, arising from his distorted sexual development, are the source of his behavioral difficulties. The formulation categories now seem to be a mixture of transactional and psychodynamic. The new information requires a change in the treatment plan, since the original plan was based on a false premise. In particular, she must switch from an exploratory to a directive strategy.

George says he is unwilling to leave her care and he also rejects her suggestions of medication or a peer-support group. In negotiation, the patient has the power to say no. Fortunately, after four "regular" sessions, he has apparently formed a reasonable therapeutic alliance that promises to support her work with him. Under these circumstances Jane has decided to continue with him, but she feels pressured to provide new tactics without having prior experience with this kind of problem. She feels outside her comfort zone and rushes to fill the gap between her experience and George's need to control his impulses. Using her familiarity with cognitive-behavioral principles and George's specific history, Jane tries to use her general experience and her own creativity to craft a new treatment plan, one that is unique to this patient. Coming up with new tactics in an area she is unfamiliar with carries its own risks.

Jane finds it hard to believe George has no experience with online pornography. Concealing information is a universal human trait. Our species has successfully taken control of the entire planet, not least because of our ability to deceive, mislead, prevaricate and conceal. In short, we are all liars and this trait is as common in psychotherapy settings as it is everywhere else. So it does not surprise Jane when she hears that George has lied by omission about his most important secret, his longstanding voyeurism. She realizes she still does not have the full story. Her writing assignment is an effort to overcome his obvious resistance to telling her his past offenses in the office.

Jane uses herself as a subject for exposure and response prevention after she notices him staring at her chest. She offers herself as a sexual object while still hoping to maintain a professional reliance on her expertise. This tactic has the value of immediacy and includes her ability to directly monitor his behavior, but it is somewhat questionable. First, it risks interference with the therapeutic alliance. Second, Jane comes close to supporting a boundary violation, as she mixes this therapeutic tactic with their real relationship. Lastly, the immediacy of this task, the way it exposes George's pathology right in the office, may create a disruptive sense of humiliation and anxiety.

Her final tactic is her prescription of watching pornography in order to siphon off some of the internal pressure to engage in actual voyeuristic activity. This exercise may risk substituting one bad habit for another (Bőthe et al., 2021). It is worth noting, however, that her on-the-spot tactic has helpful parallels with George's voyeurism: it is done in secret, the watcher is unobserved, and the act of watching confers the same "power" on the pornography viewer. These similarities suggest it can substitute a legal, low risk conduct for the high risk, illegal voyeurism.

If George is able to accept these tactics, Jane can evaluate how promising his prognosis may be. Perhaps she can continue to design additional tactics. She can also research the available literature to see what else may be helpful. She can seek supervision from someone more knowledgeable about this type of problem. If her efforts are not successful, Jane can use their failure as a basis for renewing her suggestions to try medication or to find an alternative treatment program.

Jane's choice to continue with George reflects her unwillingness to abandon her client. The wisdom of this decision remains to be tested. She has no evidentiary basis for the interventions she has come up with in the session. Instead, she has called upon her general knowledge base to create a new treatment program.

## SESSION SIX

The session is scheduled for 2:00 PM. Jane sits in the office waiting for a call from the reception desk that George has arrived. After ten minutes she walks out to the waiting room and sees George is not there. She checks with the desk and is told he had been there about a half hour before and left an envelope for her. She takes the envelope back to the office and reads the note inside, which is scrawled on a piece of yellow pad paper.

> *I've decided to solve my problems on my own.*
> *Thanks for your help.*
> *George*

A client who leaves treatment early is a treatment failure. It is unusual for a client to drop out by leaving a note. Jane speculates that

George did so to assure himself that he would not be contacted again.

Jane returns to the office and considers what might have gone wrong. One factor must certainly have been George's shame about another person knowing his secret sexual compulsion. He only revealed it under the stress of his experience with the police arriving in the midst of his rooftop spying. Perhaps that fear was diminished by his confession to her and once he left the office he felt reassured enough that he regretted telling Jane about his behavior.

Jane wonders if the problem was her revised treatment plan. His initial willingness to stay with her may have dissipated in the face of her difficult (for him) treatment requirements. Was she too aggressive in her prescriptions: making herself the focus of one exercise and, for another, suggesting pornography as a substitute outlet for him? Or perhaps it was her assignment that he write down and show her all of his past voyeuristic episodes, given how reluctant he was to reveal them in the session. Perhaps he had no intention of following her plan, but pretended to go along with it. She has no way of finding out, of course, and George may have had other reasons for his decision.

Whatever George's reasons for dropping out might have been, the underlying cause was the apparent relative weakness of the therapeutic alliance. Evidently, it was not as solid as Jane believed. In fact, almost always when a client leaves therapy prematurely the reasons will usually include a weak alliance, either because of gradual deterioration in the relationship over time or a sudden breach due to some breakdown in the treatment plan (Sharf et al., 2010). The next time George comes to official attention may be because he has been caught peeping and arrested. If he is ordered into treatment by the judicial system, a positive outcome will be unlikely.

Jane decides to send him a formal letter acknowledging his decision to leave treatment and offering again to facilitate his finding an alternative program or therapist, as well as reminding him that, if he changes his mind, she will see him again herself. Such a letter not only recognizes Georges' legal jeopardy but also serves to protect Jane from any legal consequences herself. Her letter will memorialize the decision to leave therapy as George's decision alone and establishes that she did not abandon him.[4] Since she has the rest of George's session time available she drafts the letter:

Dear George,

This letter will confirm your decision today to discontinue your treatment with me here at the Student Health Service against my advice. I strongly recommend that you continue to seek help elsewhere and I would be glad to suggest other providers. Or, if you wish to continue with me, we could resume our work.

Please let me know if I can be of further help.

## Notes

1  A legal duty to warn, which requires a breach of confidentiality, varies among jurisdictions. Some states require notice to the intended victim if a patient overtly threatens another person. Others merely provide a legal shield if the therapist makes such a report.
2  Failure to adhere to community standards of care might be the basis for a suit.
3  The Health Insurance Portability and Accountability Act of 1996.
4  Abandonment is one of the legal bases for a malpractice suit. If a health care provider terminates the relationship without reasonable notice and does not give the patient an opportunity to find alternative care a malpractice claim can result.

## References

Bőthe, B., Tóth-Király, I., Griffiths, M. D., Potenza, M. N., Orosz, G., & Demetrovics, Z. (2021). Are sexual functioning problems associated with frequent pornography use and/or problematic pornography use? Results from a large community survey including males and females. *Addictive Behaviors*, 112, 106603.

Fadjukoff, P., Pulkkinen, L., & Kokko, K. (2016). Identity formation in adulthood: A longitudinal study from age 27 to 50. *Identity*, 16(1), 8–23.

Sharf, J., Primavera, L. H., & Diener, M. J. (2010). Dropout and therapeutic alliance: A meta-analysis of adult individual psychotherapy. *Psychotherapy: Theory, Research, Practice, Training*, 47(4), 637–645.

# Ellen

## A Nurse in a High Stress Job

### Referral

Ellen is a private client referred by her primary care provider, an APRN, whom she consulted for "anxiety," which worsened after she received a disciplinary warning at work (for lateness) and feared she might be fired. Her APRN prescribed Ativan and sent her to Jane.

Jane sees Ellen in her private office where she and her three partners practice. They occupy the second floor of an old house converted to professional offices. The building is owned by an internist whose rooms are on the ground floor. Jane's office has a large window overlooking the rear of the building. Inside, her desk and files take up the back half of the room. In the middle she has her own chair next to a small table. Two patient chairs, flanking another small table, set with a box of tissues, are placed about eight feet across from her. A yellow and gray oval rug covers the floor in this sitting area. Table lamps are available to augment the illumination from the window. During afternoon appointments, however, sunshine through the window gives the room a cheery glow.

### History

Ellen's chief complaint is "I'm always worried and it's affecting my whole existence." She wants to get control of her life and hopes therapy can help her do so.

She is a 50 year old registered nurse who is employed on the psychiatry service of a large hospital system. Although she has worked in psychiatry throughout her career, she has only been at

DOI: 10.4324/9781003353003-6

her current job for four years. Six months earlier a new manager took over at her unit. Ellen calls her a "corporate flunky" because the woman seems more concerned with the budget than with her staff. She mismanages staffing schedules, frequently leaves the unit understaffed ("saving money") and appears indifferent to staff problems. Ellen has had trouble getting herself to work and employee lateness incurs disciplinary "points" which she fears will lead to her termination. Outside of work, she has been short-tempered, overeating and oversleeping. She feels trapped: there are no other jobs for someone with her skills and experience in this part of the state—her hospital has bought up every practice and smaller hospital in their expanding corporate empire—and she could not get equivalent salary and benefits elsewhere.

Ellen married at 23 and has two children. Her daughter, 25, works as a medical assistant in a primary care office. Her 22 year old son graduated from the State university but is so far unemployed and living with her in her two bedroom condominium. Ellen divorced her husband ten years ago after she discovered he was being unfaithful. She has not dated since the divorce and has no plans to "start all that crap all over again."

## Mental Status Examination

Ellen arrived at the initial interview in her hospital uniform. Her overall presentation was one of controlled anger as she spoke of her resentment at her treatment at work and her frustration that she was stuck in her job. She expressed feeling helpless about her "no win" situation and cried when she discussed it. She described her mood as irritable rather than hopeless and denied suicidal ideation. Notable personality traits include an overdeveloped need for control and a tendency toward perfectionism.

## Formulation

Ellen's professional skills and experience have failed to protect her against the strains created by an unfavorable work environment. Since she has relied on these abilities throughout her adult life, she is limited now in finding new ways to deal with these stresses. As noted, she is somewhat rigid and perfectionistic, with an overdeveloped need for control, traits that have been helpful in her profession, but now may aggravate her difficulties with the new management. Her current difficulties fall into the category of situational stress: her personality traits and skill set clash with the requirements of a flawed work environment.

Ellen has done well in earlier jobs and presumably she would again if the adverse factors in her current job were to disappear. Since that appears unlikely, and because the difficulties in adapting to the new conditions now threaten to get her fired, her only option is to change her behavior in ways that minimize the existing conflicts. Jane suspects, however, that her rigid personality and her self-righteous feeling of injustice will make change difficult. Significant personality modifications will be challenging given her age and resources, although she may be able to soften them if convinced it is necessary. The more productive area on which to focus may be to use her existing skills to better handle her job problems. Her motivation for therapy is high. Her motivation for change is moderate.

(Formulation Category: Situational)

## Treatment Plan

Jane hopes she can help Ellen mobilize her considerable skills and experience to manage her work problems more successfully while also somewhat modifying the role her personality traits play in aggravating them. She decides a reasonable *aim* of her work with Ellen is increased psychological flexibility.

The main *goal* must be to help Ellen adapt to the difficult work environment. A secondary *goal* is to moderate her overdeveloped traits to the degree that she can function better in her day to day job on the psychiatric unit. If she succeeds with this goal she expects Ellen will find more satisfaction in her clinical work.

Jane expects to use a cognitive-behavioral *strategy* to deal with the cognitive distortions that underlie Ellen's perception and response to her work environment. She suspects she may also need some psychodynamic interventions to help Ellen modify her poorly adaptive personality traits, a challenging task under the best of circumstances, although it is possible that Ellen's situation will improve without those changes.

## Treatment Contract

Jane proposes to Ellen that they use their time together to find new ways to deal with the job problems and especially those that threaten her employment status. Ellen appears skeptical. She says, "It's not me. It's them." and Jane replies that "they" are not in the room and the only person who can solve the problem is Ellen herself. After some discussion of this fact, Ellen remains skeptical but agrees to "give it a try."

## SESSION THREE

After the initial interview, the next session (Session Two) was taken up with Ellen venting her frustration and resentment about how badly the ward is run, her clashes with her coworkers, her disappointment at the lack of support from her manager, and other job-related complaints. Jane listened to this CHRONICLE of complaints without trying to intervene because of the pressured speech and emotional intensity behind the words, but she hopes that she can use today's session to bring the focus onto their therapy goals.

Ellen arrives today in her nurse's uniform with RN embroidered on the loose blue tunic, having come just after her shift. She looks tired and somewhat disheveled.

Time remaining
45 minutes

Ellen            (Slumps in her chair) What a day! They had us short-staffed and we had four admissions and three discharges. One of the patients had to go to the ER and I had to send a staff with her which left us even more short-handed…

Jane          (Raises her hand, palm out) Ellen, I want to bring up
              an issue with you about how we're using our time to
              work on your problems.

              *Jane uses a strong hand gesture to*
              *demonstrate the significance of this*
              *interruption. She elects to address Ellen by*
              *her first name in order to personalize and*
              *emphasize the importance of what she wants*
              *to say. Since Jane introduced herself to*
              *Ellen by her last name, this disparity could*
              *undermine the* THERAPEUTIC ALLIANCE *by*
              *implying a parent-child relationship, or sound*
              *condescending or even demeaning. Jane knows*
              *that most people call her "Ellie," however, so*
              *the use of her more formal name is less risky.*

Ellen         (Sits up) Did I do something wrong?

Jane          No, not wrong, but maybe not helpful. It's just that
              we've been spending our time reviewing the kinds of
              problems you're having at work instead of looking
              for ways to improve things. You come in with a lot of
              stuff to tell me, like today, about being short-handed
              and swamped. Wouldn't we be better off figuring out
              how to solve these problems instead of you just tell-
              ing me about them?

              *Ellen responds as if she is at fault ("Did I*
              *do something wrong?"), demonstrating a*
              *vulnerability to perceived criticism. Jane*
              *files away that observation as something to*
              *deal with at a future time. She does not want*
              *to distract the discussion from the current*
              *topic. Jane alludes to the problem without*
              NAMING *it ("*CHRONICLING*") because Ellen*
              *would feel more criticized. Instead, she*

> *merely cites an example and carefully labels*
> *it "not helpful" instead of "wrong."*

Ellen    (Frowns) So I shouldn't tell you about work? That's why I'm here, isn't it?

Jane    Not exactly. We're here to look for ways for you to deal with the work problems, not just to get them off your chest. If all you needed was to hash over what's going on at work, you wouldn't need me to do it.

> *Jane restates the issue bluntly to emphasize*
> *the weight of the problem. (Ellen uses "I"*
> *while Jane uses "we" to emphasize the need*
> *for collaboration.)*

Ellen    (Whining) But I feel better when I get it all out here. I don't have anybody else who'd listen the way you do.

Jane    Yes, but isn't that just a temporary solution? Sure, you feel better when you leave here but nothing changes and the next time you'll have another list of grievances to tell me.

> *Ellen ignores Jane's invitation to look for*
> *ways to improve and restates her position.*
> *She's not ready to give up on using Jane's*
> *sympathetic shoulder to unload on. In*
> *effect, they are renegotiating the TREATMENT*
> *CONTRACT, which now looks like a false*
> *agreement. Ellen **wants** a sympathetic*
> *listener and Jane **wants** to look for solutions.*
> *Unless they agree on a single "want," this*
> *therapy will end in an IMPASSE or in Ellen*
> *dropping out. Jane rejects Ellen's version of*
> *the contract with no room for compromise.*
> *She uses the word "grievance," a term*

*common in employee–employer relation
conflicts, to suggest that Ellen is making a
job-related problem into a personal problem.
In other words, she tries to* RENAME *the
problem in a more concrete way that may
make it easier to discuss.*

Ellen    (Bitterly) So, I'm just a loud-mouth complainer.

Jane    If complaining was all the therapy was about you
wouldn't need a therapist.

> *In response to Jane's refusal to consider
> Ellen's treatment plan ("I'll complain;
> you listen") Ellen makes another defensive
> statement. By negatively exaggerating what
> Jane said, Ellen tries to deflect the discussion.
> If Jane took the bait, she would have to explain
> herself, deny that she's criticizing, and so on,
> all of which would stymie the dialogue of how
> to use therapy more successfully. Jane ignores
> the exaggeration, picks up Ellen's negative
> word ("complainer"), and restates her initial
> observation.*

Ellen    (Warily) So what do you want me to do?

Jane    I'd like us to try, together, to see how you can cope
with these work problems more successfully. We could
start by taking one of your issues and talking about how
you're handling it and how you could do better.

> *Ellen indicates that she might accept
> the contract, but says "me," not "us,"
> suggesting that the* THERAPEUTIC ALLIANCE
> *may be at stake here. Jane emphasizes the
> collaborative basis she wants (she again
> uses "we") and restates the treatment* GOAL,

*adding a specific invitation to make the idea*
*more concrete.*

Ellen    (Throws up her hands) Pick one? How about the short staffing. What do you think I should do about that? I can't get more staff in. I have to work with what they give me.

Jane    That's a good point. You and I, sitting here, can't make your unit run any better. We can't improve the staffing. We can't change the kind of inappropriate patients they admit. We can't make your corporate flunky be a better manager. All we can do is look at what **you** do and see whether there are better ways to handle things.

> *Ellen suggests that Jane's idea is ridiculous.*
> *She is not ready to accept the* TREATMENT PLAN.
> *Jane acknowledges the reality of her work*
> *issues. She repeats Ellen's pejorative term for*
> *her manager ("corporate flunky"), a use of*
> DICTION, *to show she is on Ellen's side. She*
> *then uses it to make the important point that*
> *the therapy* AIM *is to change Ellen's behavior.*

Ellen    So, like what?

> Time remaining
> 35 minutes

Jane    Well, for instance, what if we start with you checking in late and getting those points against your record? Isn't that the biggest threat right now? Possibly getting fired?

> *Ellen seems to recognize the truth of Jane's*
> *explanation and its consequences. Jane picks*
> *the most important behavior, the one that*

*threatens Ellen's job and requires a behavior change most urgently. Jane accepts her inquiry of what to work on as a tacit acceptance of the clarified contract and hopes they can continue on that new basis. She asks questions rather than make resistance-producing statements about what to work on.*

Ellen    Yeah, they fired one of the mental health workers last week 'cause he was falling asleep on the job. Poor guy was working three jobs and he couldn't help himself.

Jane    So it's a real threat.

> *She emphasizes the importance of this problematic behavior.*

Ellen    (Soberly) Yeah, it is.

Jane    Did you always have trouble with time management or did it start more recently?

> *NAMING the problem "time management," a neutral term (instead of the more critical and inflammatory "ACTING OUT," a phrase Ellen would recognize from her own training) is a first step in getting her to focus on the issue.*

Ellen    Well, not always, but I've never been one to be ahead of the game when it comes to keeping track of my time.

Jane    And when did you start getting points for lateness?

> *Ellen accepts the new label. Jane asks for details to establish a FOUNDATION for finding a solution.*

| Ellen | (Thinking back) I'd say it's been the last three months. |
|---|---|

| Jane | And what was going on three months ago? |
|---|---|

*Ellen begins to cooperate with the idea of examining her own behavior. Analyzing the origin of a behavior requires a detailed understanding of the ANTECEDENTS and DYNAMICS surrounding its inception.*

| Ellen | Oh, I think it was my vacation request. I wanted time off the week of Labor Day because it's my son's birthday and also I wanted to use four days and have the holiday for the fifth day. I put the request in early, in January! And I should have gotten it. But when the schedule came out my time off wasn't on it. |
|---|---|

| Jane | Did you do anything about it? Talk to your manager? |
|---|---|

*She asks for more details, a prerequisite to constructing a better response for Ellen. "Talk to your manager" is also a subtle reference to a behavior that is not ACTING OUT.*

| Ellen | I sent her an email but it didn't matter. Nothing changed. |
|---|---|

| Jane | So you felt, what? Disappointed? Angry? Abused? |
|---|---|

*Jane wants to focus on Ellen's feelings as well as facts. She NAMES three possibilities.*

| Ellen | "Abused." (Shakes her head) Yeah, I did. That's the way they treat us at that place. Expect us to do everything for them and they do nothing for us. All they care about is making more money. Fill the beds. |
|---|---|

| Jane | You're still angry about it. |
|---|---|

*Ellen airs her grievances again but now it's in the service of dealing with the problem. With this METACOMMUNICATION Jane NAMES her feeling, laying a FOUNDATION for pointing out how Ellen's ACTING OUT has been ineffective and possibly harmful, if it gets her fired.*

Ellen        Damn right I am.

Jane         So you started coming in late.

*She makes a specific connection between the anger and the ACTING OUT. A question would risk less resistance than this statement, such as "Do you think being angry was what made you start coming in late?"*

Ellen        (Raised eyebrows) I don't plan to be late! Some days I have trouble just getting myself out the door. I keep doing other things until the last minute. Then if there's traffic or something I'll be a minute or so late getting to the time clock to sign in. And it doesn't matter if you're 30 seconds late or 30 minutes late; they hit you with the points.

Jane         "They hit you." Sounds like you feel this points system is an attack.

*Predictably, Ellen does resist Jane's statement. Instead, she blames external sources for her lateness, like the traffic. Jane tries another approach. If Ellen feels attacked, she might feel her behavior is justified, even though her lateness hurts her more than her manager. Jane's focus here is getting Ellen to accept her responsibility for the problem and therefore her ability to solve it.*

Ellen    Well, it is. I mean, in most jobs if you're late getting in you can make it up on the other end, stay past quitting time. At this hospital if you do clock out late you get even more points!

Jane    I agree. That is abusive.

*The* THERAPEUTIC ALLIANCE *has been weakened by Jane's challenge to her behavior. In spite of the risk of agreeing with the client's perspective (which may not be the reality of the situation), Jane* NAMES *the problem as "abusive" in the interest of maintaining the alliance with her. Whether or not the employer is abusive or reasonable it will still be up to Ellen to find a solution.*

Ellen    I'm glad you think so. Before, it sounded like you were on their side.

Jane    It's not a matter of taking sides. It's a question of what's the best thing to do about it.

*Ellen's comment about being "on their side" confirms the threat to the* THERAPEUTIC ALLIANCE. *Still, Jane doesn't say, "No, I'm on your side," since that would imply that she approves of Ellen's* ACTING OUT. *Instead she restates the treatment* GOAL.

Ellen    (Skeptically) Yeah, and what's that?

Jane    Let's hear what you think.

*Jane avoids the temptation to tell her to show up on time as a start, and thereby take on the role of "wise problem-solver" so Ellen doesn't need to be responsible for her behavior. Instead, she invites her collaboration.*

Ellen        I think I should find somewhere else to work, but
             that's not possible. I'd have to give up all my ben-
             efits, my pension, and no place else around here has
             openings that would pay me what I'm getting. I'm
             stuck.

Jane         I see that.

             *She acknowledges the reality of Ellen's
             dilemma. Again, Jane wants to keep the
             THERAPEUTIC ALLIANCE intact.*

Ellen        So what should I do?

                                                  Time remaining
                                                  25 minutes

Jane         The question is, is arriving late doing anything to solve
             the problem, and, if not, what else could you do?

             *Ellen takes Jane's agreement to mean Jane
             will have the answer for her. Jane is careful
             to avoid becoming the problem-solver.
             Instead, her question reiterates her stance
             that Ellen needs to find a way to change.*

Ellen        Well, obviously, being late is making things worse.
             I'll have to do better. (Shrugs) Get there on time.

Jane         That would be a start. But is there a better way to han-
             dle your anger at the manager or, really, at the whole
             system?

             *She acknowledges Ellen's resolution to be
             on time, but then emphasizes the general
             problem of anger management that caused
             her to be late. Without saying it overtly she
             has now RENAMED the neutral term, "time*

*management," as the more accurate anger target, hospital management.*

Ellen    (Shakes her head) You got me. I don't know.

Jane    Well, let's think about this: behind all the problems you see at work seems to be your expectation that things should be working better. What I mean is, you're measuring the place against your standards of what a well-run, efficient, effective unit should be. The ideal unit, where, for instance, people get the time off they deserve.

> *Ellen counters with another defensive statement, as if Jane was giving her a test rather than inviting her to work together on a solution. Jane introduces the idea that one of Ellen's personality traits—perfectionism—might shape her behavior at work.*

Ellen    That is what I expect. (Pauses) Well, maybe not ideal but certainly better than what's there. What's wrong with that?

Jane    Based on what you've told me about the corporation that runs the hospital and the type of management you've described, is it realistic to think that the place could change for the better? Is there any evidence that they're even trying to improve? In fact, they might think there's nothing to improve. Maybe they like it just the way it is.

> *Ellen doesn't view her expectations as unrealistic: if she expects things to be perfect, she assumes that everyone would agree with her. Her perfectionistic trait is EGO SYNTONIC. Jane indirectly restates her premise that she and Ellen cannot change anything*

*except Ellen's own behavior. Repetition, or
WORKING THROUGH, is usually needed before
a client can modify their behavior.*

Ellen    (Nods) You know, I think that's right. They're always
boasting about what a great place it is.

Jane    So, if it's never going to change, then perhaps you
need to change your expectations and act accordingly.

*Ellen begins to accept Jane's premise. Jane
now states her proposal directly.*

Ellen    You think I should just do the minimum and collect
my paycheck?

Jane    Isn't that what other employees are doing?

*Ellen makes an all-or-nothing comment
that avoids looking for a way she can
change. Jane has not said or implied she
should not do her best. Jane's question
comes uncomfortably close to giving the
advice that Jane wants to avoid, even
though she is tempted to just tell her client
what to do.*

Ellen    (Frowns) Yeah. Drives me crazy.

Jane    So that's not the answer.

*Fortunately, Ellen doesn't take Jane's
question as a prescription but instead reverts
to her "ideal" view of the service, one where
everybody works to their full ability. Jane
backtracks from her near-advice.*

Ellen    No.

Jane        So, then what?

            *She wants to shift the problem back to her*
            *client.*

Ellen       (Shrugs) I'll just have to make myself get there on
            time.

Jane        How will you do that?

            *Now that Ellen has come up with an idea*
            *on her own, Jane wants to reinforce the*
            *accomplishment. At the same time, a mere*
            *resolution may not be successful unless Ellen*
            *makes a behavioral change to put it into*
            *effect. Her question invites Ellen to continue*
            *to take responsibility.*

Ellen       (Grimaces) I'll just do it.

Jane        I remember you said you have trouble getting out the
            door. That you're all ready to go but you start doing
            something else or you get involved somewhere else
            and then when you do leave you're already going to
            be late.

            *"I'll just do it" isn't a behavioral plan. Since*
            *Ellen seems stumped, Jane introduces a*
            *focal point for her to use.*

Ellen       Yeah. I just hate going in so much that I dawdle
            around and put it off.

Jane        What about that? Any ideas how you could get around
            that problem?

            *Ellen is now able to accept responsibility*
            *for her lateness, a major step forward. Jane*
            *again invites Ellen to be in control.*

Ellen        Maybe I should set a time to leave. You know, a deadline.

Jane         Uh-huh.

             *She has to be careful here not to take ownership of the plan. She makes a simple acknowledgement.*

Ellen        Then, if I keep an eye on that…

                                                    Time remaining
                                                    15 minutes

Jane         Yes, I see what you mean.

             *Again, she tries to encourage her without making the decision.*

Ellen        Because, you know, I'm pretty good about getting ready for work. Changing into my uniform, getting my meal packed, all that stuff. Then I fart around and next thing I know I'm going to be late.

Jane         I think you're right. That's where the problem happens.

             *She underlines the point she made earlier, that leaving for work is where the behavior is a problem.*

Ellen        Sometimes it's not my fault. Traffic is bad. I get behind a school bus. It just takes longer some days than others.

Jane         Can you build that into your plan? Maybe leave early enough that bad traffic won't make you late?

             *Ellen backs away from the plan to change her behavior by citing factors (traffic jams, school buses) she presumably can't control.*

*In other words, it's not her problem and changing won't make a difference. Jane feels frustrated. She thought they had succeeded but now it looks uncertain. Her frustration leads her to giving Ellen a solution rather than asking her to solve it.*

Ellen    But if I get there early I can't check in. You get points if you clock in ahead of time. They've got you either way.

Jane    Isn't it better to stand around and wait to check in rather than to be late and get penalized?

*Ellen, predictably, reacts to Jane's advice with a "yes, but" response of RESISTANCE. Jane responds to this comment with a question, still trying to salvage the plan. A METACOMMUNICATION here might have been more effective, something like, "It sounds like you're looking for reasons not to solve the problem."*

Ellen    (Microexpression of annoyance) I guess so.

Jane    You don't sound convinced.

*Again, a METACOMMUNICATION seems indicated.*

Ellen    I guess I hate to let them win.

Jane    Win?

*Jane recognizes that Ellen has introduced a new facet of the problem. Rebellion against authority has not specifically come up before, but it may be the reason Ellen seems to back*

*away from solving her lateness problem.*
*Unfortunately, most of the session is over.*

Ellen    They're a bunch of bullies. They have all the power, the bastards.

Jane    I see. It hurts you to let them succeed.

*All she can do now is acknowledge Ellen's*
*feelings with the METACOMMUNICATION and*
*perhaps they'll be able to work on it in the*
*next session.*

Ellen    Damn right!

Jane    But what you're saying is, if you arrive on time and leave on time then the hospital wins. Is that it? It's some kind of game?

*Jane states the reality of the job*
*requirements as a way of underlining that*
*the problem is Ellen's and therefore it's in*
*her power to change and solve it.*

Ellen    Okay, when you put it that way it sounds stupid.

Time remaining
5 minutes

Jane    Aren't you the one making it a game?

*She makes an INTERPRETATION that states*
*her premise and implies that Ellen can*
*control her behavior. By phrasing it as a*
*question, Jane hopes to have it more easily*
*accepted.*

Ellen    Me?

| | |
|---|---|
| Jane | (Cocks her head and raises her eyebrows) |
| | *Jane lets silence answer for her.* |
| Ellen | Well, yeah, when you think about it that way, I guess I am. |
| Jane | (Nods) |
| | *Again, her non-verbal response is more effective than restating her premise.* |
| Ellen | If that's the way it is, there's no way I can win. |
| Jane | Doesn't seem so. |
| | *This time an overt statement is stronger.* |
| Ellen | That doesn't make it any easier. |
| Jane | That's true. |
| | *An empathic statement that may strengthen the* THERAPEUTIC ALLIANCE. |
| Ellen | (Frowns) Shit. |
| Jane | Maybe "winning" isn't the best way to think about it. |
| | *She begins to lay a* FOUNDATION. |
| Ellen | How should I think about it? |
| Jane | When we started out talking about this lateness problem we were looking for how you might manage your time more successfully. We weren't talking about winning or losing. |
| | *She expands the* FOUNDATION *by reminding Ellen of their earlier discussion, using the neutral concept, "time management."* |

Ellen          (Shrugs) True.

Jane           And if it was a game, the stakes are much higher for you than for the hospital.

> *She now can use the FOUNDATION to make her point more strongly.*

Ellen          What do you mean?

Jane           If you get fired for too many points, who suffers the most? You're out of a job, with all the bad consequences that brings with it. The hospital just has to hire a new nurse. Not a big deal for them.

> *At the end of the session she wants to leave Ellen with a clear understanding of this idea.*

Ellen          (Raises her eyebrows) Ah, I see what you mean.

Jane           Our time is up for today and we have to stop.

> *Jane feels Ellen has accepted the idea that the solution of her work problems is up to her. She hopes using the session to air her grievances has ended and will carry over to future sessions but it may require more work in the service of WORKING IT THROUGH.*

### Discussion

Therapy stagnates when clients use their therapy time to recite their grievances, bewail the injustice of their situation and air their resentments, or when they doggedly chronicle the (therapeutically meaningless) events that have occurred since their last session. The therapy, in effect, is without a treatment plan. This misuse of their sessions can lead to "interminable" outcomes where clients continue to catalog their problems but do not modify or alter how they deal with them. The therapist can get caught up in this paradigm, resigned to listening and sympathizing without making any headway in helping these people recover.

At worst, allowing a client to use the time to complain and ask for sympathy may lead to a long-term relationship without any progress. When this happens the therapist feels comfortable with the client and gives up the idea of therapeutic change. This kind of "supportive therapy" can become a never-ending but profitable way to fill a therapy time slot.[1] That outcome would not only be unethical, it would harm the person who came for help but who instead gets a deepening dependency on the therapist.

This session was an exercise in getting a client to change a particular type of behavior by placing the responsibility for the change on her instead of giving in to the temptation to tell her what to do, appealing as that may be. Although she struggled at times, Jane resisted the easier path, knowing that if she became the problem-solver it would not lead to real success. "Give someone a fish and they'll eat for a day; teach them to fish and they'll eat for a lifetime" is the underlying idea. In the end, Ellen managed to take responsibility for her behavior. If she succeeds, her modified behavior will remove the threat that the hospital will fire her.

The work of this session operated on two levels. On one level, Jane tried to encourage Ellen to mobilize her anger at the deficiencies of hospital management to fuel a solution to her chronic lateness. At risk is the damaging consequence of merely acting out her displeasure: the loss of her job. At a deeper level, Jane tried to soften the clash between, on the one hand, Ellen's exaggerated need for control and her perfectionistic standards and, on the other hand, the reality of a poorly managed work environment that falls far short of these standards. They made progress on the immediate problem. It looks like Ellen will get to work on time. The problematic traits are ego syntonic aspects of her personality and consequently Ellen feels little motivation to deal with them. Any attempted modification would involve a change in Ellen's identity, which at this point in her life seems thoroughly settled. Nevertheless, Jane regards some softening of Ellen's rigid character as an unstated but helpful therapy goal and she will continue to look for opportunities to help her modify it.

## SESSION FOUR

Ellen hurries into the room, again wearing her hospital uniform, and sits down heavily. She appears impatient to speak as Jane settles herself across from her.

Time remaining
45 minutes

Jane          What's up?

> *Jane acknowledges her client's distress instead of waiting passively to hear what is upsetting her. Showing concern for real suffering strengthens the* THERAPEUTIC ALLIANCE.

Ellen         (Breathlessly) One of our patients attacked a nurse and broke his nose. It was… It was… I don't know. This woman, she's one of our frequent flyers. She gets readmitted every few months. (Shakes her head) She was escalating right from the start of the shift, and nobody did anything about it. No PRNs, nobody tried to redirect her, nothing, until finally she started screaming at her nurse and then hitting him. So we called a staff assist and put her in restraints, and we medicated her. But it was too late for Jason, he's the nurse she beat up. (She sinks back into her chair)

Jane          Sounds like it's a scary place to work.

> *In this* METACOMMUNICATION, *she reflects the feeling attached to the event rather than its details since it is the emotional consequences of the event that she expects Ellen will need help with.*

Ellen         (Throws up her hands) The whole thing could have been avoided if staff did their jobs.

Jane        It was the fault of the staff?

            *She wonders why Ellen doesn't blame the*
            *assaultive patient. Asking the question*
            *confronts Ellen with the apparent distortion.*

Ellen       This shit wouldn't happen if people did their jobs! If
            the hospital cared about staff instead of taking any-
            body who shows up just to fill the beds and keep the
            bucks rolling in.

Jane        What happened to the patient? Did they call the
            police?

            *Jane's curiosity overcomes her treatment*
            *STRATEGY as she asks for more facts. A better*
            *response would have been to zero in on*
            *Ellen's fear for her own safety. Sometimes*
            *an unusual event can lead to more progress*
            *toward therapy GOALS.*

Ellen       (Snorts) In your dreams. The hospital doesn't care
            if we get hurt. They tell us it's all part of our job.
            Nobody gives a damn and the police wouldn't do
            anything anyway. Half these people, the police bring
            them to the ER and dump 'em there. Saves them the
            paperwork and hassle if they arrested them in the first
            place. We sent Jason to the ER and now he's off for
            who knows how long on a medical.

Jane        What about you? What did all this do to your feelings
            about the unit?

            *Now she returns her attention to Ellen's*
            *emotional response.*

Ellen       (Throws up her hands) It's like I've been telling you.
            It's a shitty job and I'm stuck there.

Jane          Do you feel personally unsafe? Vulnerable?

              *Ellen prefers to discuss the work environment
              rather than her own feelings. Jane NAMES two
              possibilities as she tries to redirect her.*

Ellen         I take precautions. I never turn my back on a patient.
              I even carry a sharp-pointed pen in case I need a
              weapon. But, yeah, when somebody gets hurt it
              makes you nervous.

Jane          Are you nervous because you don't feel you're in
              control there?

              *Jane mirrors her word, "nervous," for
              the DICTION, instead of using stronger
              terms, such as fearful, insecure or angry.
              She realizes the lack of control is more
              important to Ellen than her emotional
              response to the attack. She elects to follow
              Ellen's lead and initiates a discussion of
              her need for control.*

Ellen         (Leans forward) I'm not in control. The whole unit
              gets out of control.

Jane          But you, personally, isn't that part of the problem?
              That you can't control things when you think you
              should be able to?

              *She wants to keep Ellen's attention on
              herself, not the job.*

Ellen         (Annoyed) You make it sound like it's wrong to want
              to be in control.

Jane          I'm not saying it's wrong, but isn't it a matter of degree?

*She begins to lay a FOUNDATION for
a discussion of how the trait might be
problematic. A more direct approach would
have been to challenge Ellen with the failure
of her usual efforts to control her environment.
Perhaps saying, "How's that working out for
you?" Jane feels that directly confronting Ellen
with her failure would generate resentment and
damage the THERAPEUTIC ALLIANCE, so she opts
for the gentler response. Even better would be
a METACOMMUNICATION: "Aren't you saying
you want more control than is possible in that
place?"*

Ellen        What do you mean?

Jane         How important is it to you to be in control?

*She uses a question to help Ellen think about
it rather than looking to Jane to explain it.*

Ellen        (Frowns) Look, there's certain ways to do things,
to do them the right way, and that's all I'm saying
I want. If that's being in control, then that's what I
want. You make it sound like it's a problem.

Jane         But isn't it a question of proportion? Things happen that you can't control, that maybe nobody could.
That's life, isn't it. Shit happens? Do you want **more**
control than it's possible for any one person to have?

*Ellen strongly resists the idea Jane has put
forward. Her need for control is an EGO
SYNTONIC trait. When Ellen normalizes her
behavior Jane has to suggest that Ellen's
need for control is excessive. Until Ellen
recognizes the abnormality of this trait (until*

*it becomes EGO DYSTONIC) she will not be able to modify it. Jane uses Ellen's DICTION ("shit happens") to promote agreement.*

Ellen    That's what you think?

Jane    That's what I'm asking you.

*She declines to become the "authority" whose opinion might be disputed or rejected. If Ellen reaches a conclusion herself she is more likely to accept it. Indirectly, however, it is obvious that Jane thinks Ellen's need for control is excessive and a problem.*

Ellen    (Reluctantly) I guess that's possible. So, what can I do about it?

Time remaining
35 minutes

Jane    What do you think?

*"I guess" suggests Ellen is not quite ready to acknowledge her greater need for control. Jane declines again to be the expert.*

Ellen    (Frowning) What do I think? I think I want to work in a safe place and not have to worry somebody's going to assault me.

Jane    And if you had more control where you work, that would make it safer?

*Ellen normalizes her need for control, showing she has not accepted it as a problem. Jane builds on the FOUNDATION she began earlier.*

Ellen    (Loudly) Damn right!

| Jane | From what you tell me about the hospital, though, it sounds like you won't be able to control it. You don't have the authority and, according to you, nobody else sees the problems you do and nobody cares enough to make things better. Now, if that's true, if you yourself can't change the way the place is run, **and** you don't want to give up the job, doesn't that mean that **you** have to change to adapt to those conditions? |

*Now she can contrast Ellen's need for control with the reality of her status as an employee.*

| Ellen | I guess, yeah, when you put it that way. |

| Jane | So. Any ideas? |

*Another "I guess." Her reluctance continues. Jane asks Ellen to strategize about the work environment. This general question deflects the discussion from Ellen's need for control. A better question might have been along the lines of: "If you need more control than the average person, how do you think you got that way?" That might lead to historical information that could help convince Ellen that a part of herself she is proud of could also be the source of her current difficulty.*

| Ellen | (Frowns) The only thing I can think of, I could be the charge nurse. That would give me some control over the unit. |

| Jane | What about that? |

*Having started down that path, she now has to pursue Ellen's ideas about her work environment.*

Ellen       (She shivers dramatically) I never want to be charge. I only take it when I'm forced to.

Jane        When you're **forced** to?

            *She repeats part of Ellen's statement with emphasis to avoid asking a "why" question.*

Ellen       Yeah, I hate it when I have to be charge. I have to give out the assignments and nobody likes their assignment. If something goes wrong they always blame me, whether it's my fault or not. That's the way that whole place runs. Something goes wrong and everybody starts pointing fingers at everybody else and when they can't blame anybody else, they blame the nurse. Doctor makes a mistake, blame the nurse. Patients go wrong, blame the nurse. Anything bad happens, blame the nurse.

Jane        Even if that's true, aren't you still better off being the one in charge? Isn't that still an advantage?

            *Jane implies that Ellen's need for control could be satisfied if she, in fact, took control of the unit. A better response might have been a METACOMMUNICATION about how helpless and vulnerable Ellen feels at work.*

Ellen       Only a little.

Jane        Hmm.

            *The same METACOMMUNICATION could help here.*

Ellen       But I see what you're getting at. A little control is better than no control.

Jane    That still leaves us with the bigger question.

> *Ellen's grudging agreement suggests she is going along with Jane's idea, but is not fully aboard. Recognizing the lost focus, Jane begins to shift it back to Ellen.*

Ellen    What's that?

Jane    Whether your need for control is excessive and that contributes to your stress. If you're the kind of person who has a strong need for control, and you're in a situation where that much control isn't possible, can you modify your own feelings so you won't be as frustrated by the mismatch?

> *Jane tries to REFRAME Ellen's need for control as EGO DYSTONIC by using the word "excessive." This statement encapsulates one of the treatment GOALS but it also is a suggestion in the form of a question.*

Ellen    (Exasperated) I can't change how I feel!

Jane    No, you can't change your feelings, but you can adjust how you act on them. That's what the therapy is all about: changing yourself to make things better for you.

> *Jane makes a direct "suggestion," one that is unlikely to modify Ellen's overdeveloped need for control. Ellen has not accepted that her need for control is a problem. Jane restates the GOAL as "changing yourself," but she's stuck with having said Ellen should "adjust" her actions.*

Ellen    So I'd still have the feelings, but I wouldn't do anything about them? That sounds impossible.

Jane            Hard, maybe. Not impossible.

                *She now must urge Ellen to make a change.*
                *Jane has undermined her own plan by giving*
                *in to the temptation to give advice.*

Ellen           I don't know if I can do that.

Jane            Let's give it a try. See how it goes.

                *Jane finds that now she has to exhort Ellen*
                *to make a change, a common pitfall when*
                *giving advice. It is unlikely to be successful*
                *and may even have the opposite effect and*
                *stiffen the client's resistance.*

Ellen           I don't know where to start.

Jane            Can you think of one thing you can change at work?

                *Jane is now invested in the plan and Ellen,*
                *unable (or unwilling) to think of a change,*
                *forces Jane to think for her.*

Ellen           (Shakes her head) One thing... Okay, I could stick
                with my patients and not bother about the rest of the
                unit.

Jane            How would that work?

                *Jane has to accept Ellen's idea and asks for*
                *details.*

Ellen           Well, whoever's in charge divides the patients up
                among the nurses on that shift. So I might have seven
                patients, Jason might have the same and whoever

else is on would get seven and the charge would take the rest. We each give out the meds to our group of patients and take care of whatever else in the treatment plan. Ha, assuming there even is an actual treatment plan and not some boilerplate shit that doesn't mean anything.

Jane   So you might have seven patients and you're not responsible for the rest of them?

*She highlights the part of Ellen's description that includes what she might work on, rather than let her go off into a rant about what's wrong with the hospital.*

Ellen   Yeah, but it doesn't really work that way.

Jane   No?

Ellen   No. If a milieu counselor or a social worker has a question or a problem with a patient they grab the first nurse that's handy to deal with it. God forbid they should figure out the answer on their own. What I'm saying is I could refuse to go along with that. I could tell them, "Go ask **your** nurse." Go ask the nurse in charge of that patient.

Jane   I see.

*Again, she supports the focus on the specific problem.*

Ellen   But that's only part of it. Because when I see something wrong, even if it's not my patient, I try to take care of it. I mean, if I know what to do and nobody else is willing to act, then I tend to take over when I really shouldn't have to.

Jane          Things you're not responsible for.

              *Rather than a problem, Ellen sees her behavior*
              *as an asset. Jane introduces a focus on another*
              *problematic trait, that Ellen tends to be overly*
              *responsible, another effort at REFRAMING.*

Ellen         Exactly. But maybe I can stop doing that.

Jane          It would be interesting to see if lightening your load
              like that would lower your stress level at work.

              *Ellen's "maybe" means she acknowledges*
              *her agency but she doesn't commit to*
              *the change. An underlying problem is*
              *developing: Ellen seems willing to agree with*
              *what she thinks Jane wants without actually*
              *committing to carry it out. This discrepancy*
              *may indicate an emerging TRANSFERENCE*
              *problem, where Ellen seems to obey her*
              *"parent" but does not carry out what she*
              *sees as an order. Since her attitude has not*
              *fully surfaced or demonstrably impacted the*
              *therapy, Jane cannot address it now.*

Ellen         Uh-huh.

                                              Time remaining
                                              15 minutes

Jane          I'll look forward to hearing how that goes. Meanwhile,
              how are things going in the rest of your life?

              *Jane recognizes that Ellen's "uh-huh"*
              *doesn't commit her to change. Having come*
              *to a stalemate with this misdirected effort,*
              *Jane wisely chooses to leave it for now. A*
              *better topic would be the important problem*

*from the previous session; namely, Ellen's lateness and the threat it carries for losing her job. Instead, she asks Ellen for another problem. The "advice" struggle has thrown her off her stride.*

Ellen    (Shrugs) My son still has no job. He's basically lying around, sponging off of me. I keep pushing him to find something, but he says there's nothing available for him.

Jane    You're "pushing him?"

*She picks up on the hint of conflict between Ellen and her son. The topic of her son's job-seeking is a rather minor issue. It's as if they both silently agreed to coast through the rest of the session.*

Ellen    I'm trying to motivate him. He graduated eight months ago. It's time for him to move on.

Jane    How is he to live with?

*She wants to know the extent of the possible conflict.*

Ellen    Oh, that part's fine. He helps out. Does some shopping for me. He's got his own room. He'll even make a meal sometimes.

Jane    What kind of job does he want?

*Jane's further interest in this fairly minor subject is a telling demonstration of her frustration with Ellen's resistance to the prior topic. She asks for specifics to lay a FOUNDATION for exploring the conflict.*

| | |
|---|---|
| Ellen | Beats me. Something easy and high paid, I'd guess. He's got his student loans to pay off, so he needs something soon. |
| Jane | So, you can't control him either.<br>*The comment ("easy and high paid") suggests a lack of respect for him. Jane decides to once again introduce the need for control in this new situation.* |
| Ellen | Ha. You got that right. |
| Jane | Same problem at home as at work.<br>*She underlines it.* |
| Ellen | Yeah, but I got to do something with him. I can't let him flounder around like that. |
| Jane | What does he tell you? Does he think he's floundering?<br>*She asks for more data to help her analyze the situation.* |
| Ellen | No. He says it's the tough job market. I think that's just an excuse. |
| Jane | Sounds like he doesn't want your help.<br>*Her comment tries to refine the conflict.* |
| Ellen | He's my son. It's my job to help him when I can.<br>*She cites duty, not love for her son. Jane might learn more about their relationship if she points this out.* |
| Jane | Another job where you can't control things. |

*Instead, she makes an initial*
*INTERPRETATION; namely, that it is Ellen's*
*overdeveloped personality trait that creates*
*the problem with her son.*

Ellen       When you put it that way, yeah.

Jane        Can you tell me more about him? How old is he now?
            What's he like?

            *With Ellen's apparent agreement she asks*
            *for more specifics to begin the WORKING*
            *THROUGH process.*

Ellen       He's 22. He takes after his father.

Jane        How is he like his father?

            *Ellen's former husband's behavior has not*
            *yet come up. She decides to detour a bit to*
            *find out more about him.*

Ellen       He's clever, good looking, but also kind of sneaky. I
            never really know what's he thinking. As a kid, he'd
            get into trouble and he'd try to lie his way out of it.
            We used to say he'd grow up to be a politician. You
            know, a smooth talker who never told you what he
            was really into.

Jane        So, he's like his father because he's sneaky? You've
            never said much about your former husband.

            *She diverts again to gather more history.*

Ellen       Yeah, that bastard. I dumped him a long time ago.

Jane        Wasn't that because he had an affair?

*Her choice of the word "affair" is somewhat euphemistic and may represent an error in* DICTION.

Ellen      (Irritated) An affair? He was screwing around. I found out about one of them but… Listen, he traveled a lot for work, you know? I know he had lots of "affairs" when he was on the road. I just couldn't prove it.

*Her reaction shows that the* DICTION *was off base.*

Jane      How long were you married?

*Jane moves on with taking a history. She might have learned something useful if she asked for more detail about her husband's travel and how Ellen knew what happened "on the road."*

Ellen      (Rolls her eyes) Almost 17 years.

Jane      Did it take you that long to catch on to him?

*This question could sound more critical than Jane intends. A better one would be to ask when the infidelity happened.*

Ellen      Well, he had an office job at the beginning, so if he was screwing other women I didn't know about it. He only had the job where he traveled for a few years at the end there. But it wasn't only that. When the kids were small and I was working too we needed both incomes. And also, I wanted to wait until they were older. They were in high school when we split.

Jane      It sounds like the marriage was never that great.

*Instead of a statement, a better response would be to ask a question: when did the marriage begin to be unsatisfactory?*

Ellen   At first it was. I guess that's how things go, isn't it? You're all starry eyed at the beginning and then reality sets in later. It's the usual story. I don't know what else I can tell you. He's out of my life. I don't think about him much.

Time remaining
5 minutes

Jane   Okay, getting back to your son, how does he take after his father? Is it how he treats women?

*Ellen indicates she'd like to close off the discussion, raising the question of whether she believes it's irrelevant or whether it's too painful to dredge up. Jane senses that her inquiry into the marriage is not going well and goes back to her original focus on the current problems with the son.*

Ellen   Could be. I know he goes out a lot. I don't think there's anybody special. But, then, that's how kids are these days. They don't "date" like we did. It's more of a group thing.

Jane   And he isn't married.

*"Like we did" suggests that their THERAPEUTIC ALLIANCE remains intact. Jane's response is intended to contrast the son with the husband. It implies that Ellen has invested the son with negative feelings that may be undeserved. As a FOUNDATION it may be useful for a later discussion, but it seems premature at this point.*

Ellen   No, so he's got nobody to cheat on. But give him time.

Jane   Do you think he will? Is he as untrustworthy as… what was your husband's name?

     *Nevertheless, Ellen makes the connection herself, so perhaps the comment will prove useful after all. Jane follows up on it.*

Ellen   Sam.

Jane   …as Sam was?

     *Using the man's name rather than the impersonal "your husband" may help to mobilize old emotions.*

Ellen   That sounds bad, doesn't it? It's like I'm blaming him for what his father did.

Jane   It does sound like that.

     *Ellen makes the link herself. Interpretations are usually more successful if they reflect a correlation that the client is on the verge of making already. Jane wants to reinforce her insight with a declarative agreement.*

Ellen   Maybe that's why I'm so hard on him.

Jane   You want him to get a job so he can move out. Isn't that like you're trying to divorce him, too?

     *She begins to build on Ellen's recognition of the basis for her strained relationship.*

Ellen   (Startled) Jeez, I hope not.

Jane        You hope not?

            *Repeating the phrase allows Jane to question*
            *it without using "why."*

Ellen       Well, no. I just want him to move on with his life. I'm
            not trying to get rid of him.

Jane        Okay. Well, our time is up and we have to stop.

### *Discussion*

Ellen's lateness-to-work issue occupied the therapy in the previous
session. The lateness problem is particularly important because it
threatens her job security. Jane's original plan for this session was to
follow up on the work they had done in the previous meeting. Instead,
the dangerous implications raised by a patient's assault on Ellen's fellow staff member required a shift in therapeutic focus. Ellen's personal
safety became the more pressing issue.

   Ellen works in a setting where, apparently, violence could occur
at any time and without warning. Not only was a fellow nurse seriously injured, but the apparent indifference of management ("it's all
part of the job") elevates the risk for other staff. This unfortunate trend,
where health care staff are put at risk without adequate safeguards or
back up, is a longstanding problem (Hodgkinson et al., 1985) and
it is getting worse (Stephens, 2019). Jane became caught up in the
emotional impact of the violence on Ellen's unit and her concern for
her patient's safety. As a result she found herself overly involved in
a problem-solving exercise and missed several opportunities where a
timely metacommunication might have advanced the treatment plan
more directly.

   While Jane at first tried to deal with the safety issue, Ellen
appeared to accept the danger as one of the risks of the job and was
more interested in continuing her criticism of all the ways she sees
things run badly. As a result, the discussion shifted from safety
at work to Ellen's need for control and how she could get it. Jane
initially resisted the temptation to just tell Ellen what she needed to

do, only to later begin to make suggestions. Her frustration about Ellen's resistance to change reflects the problem that personality traits are always difficult to modify and require more work than other types of behavioral problems.

Two-thirds of the way through the session, Jane abruptly switched to a different topic. This surprising and ill-advised abandonment of the issue betrayed Jane's frustration with her effort to help Ellen develop more effective coping skills. Instead of asking Ellen for another topic from "the rest of your life," Jane could more profitably have returned to the problem that occupied their last session: Ellen's chronic lateness for work and the threat that she could be fired. Instead they ended up in a review of her son's lack of a job and her divorced husband's role in the family. These topics lacked real urgency and immediacy and soon petered out as the session came to a close.

Another possibility for the slow pace of progress and for the diffi-culty Jane encountered from Ellen's resistance to helpful changes may be the covert motivation of secondary gain. Does Ellen enjoy some personal gratification from her self-image as a superior professional at the mercy of an indifferent and dangerous workplace environment? If she does, and if this is an important factor in maintaining her self-esteem, Jane will need to deal with that before she can help Ellen make significant progress toward her other goals.

This session had mixed results. On the plus side, Ellen brought up a single important topic instead of reciting a chronicle of the prior week. In the minus column is, first, Jane's diversion into the unresolved issue of taking more control through accepting the charge nurse role and, second, the failure to take up the lateness problem from the previous session. While both parties contributed to these problems, Jane was the one who could more easily have managed the agenda. Jane let her impatience with Ellen's resistance to change undercut the work she knew was needed to eventually solve these difficulties.

Future sessions are likely to follow the same pattern. Jane's efforts to focus on the underlying personality traits and the way they create unnecessary problems for Ellen will meet the resistance that arises from Ellen's rigidity and her difficulty of seeing these ego syntonic aspects of her personality as problems that need to change. These changes are not likely to yield to a short-term therapy. Jane will need patience and persistence, and a more extended treatment course, to help Ellen accommodate the demands of a difficult environment. Jane's initial decision that Ellen's problems reflected situational stress may require more focus on historical dynamics and antecedents. Ellen's therapy may need to evolve with a psychodynamic formulation focused on her maladaptive personality traits.

## Note

1 I once had a colleague who used to smugly describe these patients as "psychiatric annuities": a reliable source of income that goes on forever and requires little effort.

## References

Hodgkinson, P. E., McIvor, L., & Philips, M. (1985). Patient assaults on staff in a psychiatric hospital: A two year retrospective. *Medicine, Science and the Law*, 25(4), 288–294.

Stephens, W. (2019). Violence against healthcare workers: A rising epidemic. *The American Journal of Managed Care*, 25(5), 170–172.

# Charles

## An Older Man Facing an Existential Challenge

### Referral

Charles is self-referred, having found Jane by researching therapists online. His chief complaint is "I keep thinking about the end and it makes me wonder whether anything I do makes any difference."

### History

Charles is 75, married, with three children and five grandchildren. He retired ten years ago from his job as a certified public accountant and has been active in charity work that includes raising money for the local museum, volunteering at a homeless shelter, and working as an unpaid assistant at his local animal shelter. He plays golf and he used to breed Miniature Schnauzers, although he gave up breeding when he retired and now has only one dog as a pet. Last year he survived a Covid-19 infection. He recovered at home and he has had no continuing medical sequelae from the infection. He takes a pill for moderate hypertension. Other health problems include an enlarged prostate and arthritis. Although he has maintained his busy schedule, he has become increasingly preoccupied with fearful ruminations about aging, disability and death.

Charles grew up in the wealthy suburb of a large city and went to a small, prestigious college in a different state. He met his wife, two years younger than he, in his senior year and they married after graduation. He spent the next few years qualifying for his certificate as a CPA and then was hired by a large firm as an auditor. He

DOI: 10.4324/9781003353003-7

worked his way up and retired as an executive vice-president. His three children, a boy and two girls, are in their forties and busy with their own lives. They all live in other states, but the family comes together occasionally for special events. He describes his wife, Brenda, as a warm, supportive person who is concerned at his distress. She urged him to "seek professional help." He has no prior history of behavioral health treatment.

## Mental Status Examination

In his initial interview, Charles presented as a tall, slender man, well-groomed, wearing a three-piece suit. He had a rather stiff presentation. ("I go by Charles, not Charlie or Chuck.") He appeared mentally alert and showed no evidence of cognitive decline. He spoke softly, sat somewhat slumped in his chair and did not always make eye contact. Although he appeared sad, he denied any symptoms that would suggest a clinical depression, including suicidal ideation. In fact, although he was preoccupied with the prospect of dying, the thought of which was the identified source of his distress, he had a detached, almost emotionless, demeanor that was at odds with the content of his speech. Because of this incongruity, Jane felt both his motivation for therapy and his motivation for change were low.

## Formulation

Charles is a successful man with an accomplished history and good family support who nevertheless has been unable to face his end-of-life issues. This existential crisis interferes with his current activities and undermines his possible satisfaction with a well-earned retirement. Why someone in good health and enjoying a comfortable life should now be derailed by thoughts of his future demise is unclear to Jane from the history. She hopes to understand it better through the course of therapy and recognizes that she may have to modify her treatment plan as additional evidence emerges.

(Formulation Category: Existential)

## Treatment Plan

Jane's immediate impression of Charles is as a reserved, formal man, very much on his dignity, with a self-contained, heavily defended persona. Given the way he seems to wall off his emotions, the likelihood is that "affective experiencing"[1] will be more than usually difficult for him. She concludes that neither CBT nor a psychodynamic approach is likely to be successful because Charles will retreat into his intellectual defenses and little behavioral change will result. Jane can identify no specific target symptoms and plans to take an exploratory stance with the objective of allowing him to come to terms with his life's eventual end.

For his treatment plan, the *aim* of therapy would be "acceptance." The major *goal* would be to help Charles overcome his current affective isolation and to weaken his defensive wall sufficiently to allow an affective response to his problem. As a *strategy*, she decides to adopt a Rogerian or "client-centered" approach, a therapy considered appropriate for existential problems. Existential therapy, however, is not one of Jane's primary strengths (she usually prefers a more active approach), but she believes it could be the most effective strategy for this patient. Its primary *tactic* is to restate the patient's ideas in a way that both shows the therapist's understanding and gives the patient further insight into the meaning of his struggle. Or, as Rogers put it, "to be *with* the patient" (Rogers, 1965).

This treatment plan strikes Jane as somewhat sketchy and incomplete. Nevertheless, she feels it is a place to start and better than having no plan at all. To Charles, she says only that she will listen to his thoughts and feelings (she lays a little more emphasis on the "feelings" part) while they try to figure out, together, how Charles can cope with the stress he has been feeling. Charles looks somewhat skeptical at this proposal, but is willing to proceed and they agree on a schedule of weekly sessions. Charles dutifully records this in his iPhone. They appear to have an initial treatment contract.

## SESSION TWO

Jane is already in her private office. She opens the door and Charles enters. He again arrives in formal dress, another three-piece suit and tie, and lowers himself gingerly into one of the patient chairs.

Time remaining
45 minutes

Charles     My back is bothering me today. Must be the weather.

Jane        I'm wondering if you have any thoughts to add to what we talked about last time.

            *Jane doesn't want to have a discussion about aches and pains, at least not in this context, so she tries to redirect him to his presenting problem. It's possible that his complaint about back pain is an indirect reference to his mortality, but Jane has no evidence for this connection and if it is a covert reference it will come up again in a more discussible form.*

Charles     (Shakes his head) No new ideas. I woke up at three this morning and used the bathroom, and then I couldn't get back to sleep. A line of poetry kept going through my head. (Looks up and recites) "But at my back I always hear/ Time's wingéd chariot hurrying near;/ And yonder all before us lie/ Deserts of vast eternity."[2] Finally, I just got up and went downstairs so I wouldn't disturb Brenda.

Jane        What kept you from falling back to sleep?

            *Jane wonders at the elevated DICTION of his literary reference: Is he trying to impress her? Or sidestepping a direct expression of his*

*fears? She ignores the poem and avoids the*
*topic of his prostate problems or a discussion*
*of insomnia to focus on his mental distress.*

Charles    I was thinking that one day I would wake up dead. (Chuckles) I tried to put it out of my thoughts, but I couldn't. Once you get an idea like that in your mind it's hard to push it away. You know, it's like telling someone not to think of pink elephants.

Jane    Nothing focuses a man's mind like the prospect of being hanged in the morning?[3]

*His little laugh and his ease of recounting*
*such a scary idea suggest he is not allowing*
*any emotion associated with the idea of*
*death to come through. ISOLATION OF AFFECT*
*seems to be an important defense mechanism*
*for him, even though his fear (and his wife's*
*urging) have brought him to therapy. Jane*
*is struck by how calmly he discusses dying.*
*She tries to elicit more of a response by this*
*(mis)quote. Jane uses a quotation, a form*
*of RHETORIC, for three reasons. First, it*
*parallels Charles' intellectual presentation*
*of his reason for his troubled sleep. (His*
*voice betrays no shakiness or evidence*
*of upset.) Second, it reflects his literary*
*presentation by matching his poem with her*
*own quote; in effect, matching his DICTION.*
*Third, it restates his expressed worry*
*in a more dramatic way, as a Rogerian*
*restatement. A more active approach might*
*have been to ask him to imagine what might*
*happen in the family if they found him dead*
*in the morning, to confront the reality of his*
*death through the reactions of his family.*

| Charles | That sounds like a quote. Who said that? |
|---|---|

| Jane | I think it was Mark Twain. |
|---|---|

> *He's curious about the source but not the implication of the quote, another instance of ISOLATION OF AFFECT. She answers his question. An alternative would have been a METACOMMUNICATION; e.g., "I'm not sure who said it, but you seem awfully calm about these scary thoughts you're having. 'Waking up dead,' for instance."*

| Charles | (Nodding) Well, there's certainly truth in that. |
|---|---|

| Jane | So, then, you're feeling like you're under a death sentence? |
|---|---|

> *Jane notes the lack of emotion in his answer and tries again, with a Rogerian restatement.*

| Charles | (Raises his eyebrows) I do. When you think about it, everybody alive is under a death sentence. You're going to die; I'm going to die. We're all going to die. It's only a question of when. And odds are I'm going to die sooner. What's interesting, and I've only come to appreciate this lately, is that people don't act like death applies to them. They know it's going to happen, but only sometime in the distant future. My kids don't factor it into their lives. The grandkids don't know it even exists. I bet even somebody like you figures it's too far away, it'll never happen. |
|---|---|

| Jane | You sound frustrated. |
|---|---|

> *Now she suggests a quasi-emotional response without detailing it for him. It's both a METACOMMUNICATION and a Rogerian response.*

Charles    (Flatly) You got that right.

Jane       Can you say more about that?

           *Third try. Although what she means is more
           along the lines of "How does that make
           you feel?" Asking more directly is even less
           Rogerian than before. This approach is
           beginning to seem misguided: it's difficult to
           reflect a patient's feelings when he is not in
           touch with them.*

Charles    (Shakes his head slightly) It just puts a cloud over
           everything. I mean, you spend a lifetime accumulat-
           ing memories, knowledge and even—if I dare say
           so—wisdom, and you accomplish the things you set
           out to do. (He stops speaking and gazes out the win-
           dow) And then you die. Memories: gone. Knowledge:
           gone. Wisdom: gone. Accomplishments: gone. And
           even family and friends: all gone. I once read some-
           thing by Tolstoy where he said, "What meaning has
           life that death does not destroy?"[4] (Stares at the ceil-
           ing. His eyes appear moist.) What **meaning** has life
           that death does not destroy.

                                              Time remaining
                                              35 minutes

Jane       That your whole life is without meaning?

           *Charles answers with his own quote, using
           it to convey his feelings (as revealed by his
           sudden tearing) rather than acknowledging
           them directly. Given the hint of his feelings
           breaking through, Jane tries to keep him
           on that path, but she also responds to the
           NEGATIVE OVERGENERALIZATION by using
           "whole life" in her response, with the*

*implied question of "Is there nothing, not one single thing, in your life that has meaning for you?" She is tempted by the more active CBT TACTIC. A more Rogerian response might have been simply to agree, "Death destroys anything of value."*

Charles     Exactly. Everything I've done, it's not going to matter.

Jane        You're saying your life has been a waste of time.

*But, without the CBT TACTIC, he can agree with the idea further. He ignores the OVERGENERALIZATION idea, so Jane returns to a Rogerian restatement of his feelings.*

Charles     Well, I suppose I should recognize that my children are doing well. They seem mostly happy, although you never really know.

Jane        So, the children are your most important legacy.

*Another restatement.*

Charles     I suppose. We don't see them very much. The last time we were all together was before the pandemic. Brenda and I had our fiftieth. (Pauses, thoughtfully) They say you're never gone as long as somebody remembers you. My children and maybe the grand-kids will remember me for a while. I don't believe they'll think of me all that much. And then they'll be gone and that's the last of me.

Jane        Even the memories of your family are short-lived.

*And another restatement. But Jane is begin-ning to chafe at her passive role and she won-ders whether this approach is being helpful.*

| Charles | Yes. Think of all the billions of people who nobody remembers. It's like they never existed. The only ones who count are famous people. Mozart, Einstein... George Washington. The rest of us are just like leaves on the trees. (He waves his hands in the air) We turn brown and fall off and we're gone. We turn into dirt. |
|---|---|
| Jane | Do you think you'll know what happens after you're gone? Do you believe in an afterlife, where you might still know what's happening? |

> *Charles adds another intellectualized comment. Jane, feeling stressed by her own passivity, now begins a more active engagement with him.*

| Charles | Nah, that's a lot of crap. When you're dead, that's it. Your body rots away and there's nothing left of you. People who think otherwise are deluding themselves. |
|---|---|
| Jane | Uh-huh. |

> *He makes this distressing statement dispassionately. She hopes a simple response will encourage him to continue to speak about his death, perhaps finally tapping into his feelings.*

| Charles | You know, when I say things like that to my wife she gives me a big argument about it. You don't. Is that because you agree with me? |
|---|---|
| Jane | I don't agree or disagree. I want to get a full picture of what you're wrestling with. |

> *Instead, Charles shifts the focus to his wife and then to Jane, avoiding the implications*

*of what he just said. Jane makes a*
*temporizing statement.*

Charles      (Stares at her) Why?

Jane         Sometimes you have to put your feelings into words
             before you can really figure out how to deal with them.

             *A suggestion disguised as an educational*
             *comment. Jane is still feeling frustrated.*

Charles      (Somewhat exasperated) How can you deal with
             something like dying? It's a fact. It doesn't mat-
             ter what you tell yourself. It's not going to change
             anything.

Jane         Okay, here's another quote. Hamlet. "Nothing's
             either good or bad but thinking makes it so."[5]

             *Charles prefers intellectual debate to*
             *"putting his feelings into words." Jane uses*
             *RHETORIC to introduce a countervailing idea*
             *in the disguised form of a quotation.*

             *She continues to search for a better way*
             *to connect with him, in part by matching*
             *his DICTION (including his use of literary*
             *allusions), but she is aware that she is not*
             *having much success.*

Charles      Hamlet? I haven't seen that play. I remember reading it,
             though. A long time ago. Not sure why… Anyway, you
             believe that? It's all about how you think of something?

Jane         I see that a lot in my work.

             *"My work" is a subtle reminder that they*
             *have agreed on a task, not a mere discussion*
             *of intellectual concepts. It is also an indirect*

*way to emphasize her previous point; that his emotional response to his ideas about mortality is important to their work. Jane is caught between her decision to use the Rogerian STRATEGY and her impatience with it, since, so far, it's not helping Charles to deal with his feelings about his death.*

Charles    (Shakes his head) I don't see how death could be good, however you think about it.

Jane    Maybe not, but how you deal with the prospect, doesn't that depend on how you think about it? Or, how much you think about it?

*He's missed the point, perhaps to avoid the import of her invitation. She CLARIFIES it for him. She could have gone on to interpret his "mistake" as a defensive maneuver, but that's not in her current approach. Meanwhile, they trade quotations instead of discussing his feelings.*

Charles    Oh, I see what you mean. How I think about it. (Looks off into the distance) Yes. I'll give you an example. I have a pension that's largely held in an IRA that I manage myself. I have the money in various funds and it's doing well, so far. So, every day I tune in to one of the business channels and listen to the investment experts give out their advice on what to buy, what the market's going to do. And sometimes I hear some good ideas; like what sectors are good for the future, or specific stocks. Now, when I was younger, I might have made changes in my own portfolio based on ideas that made sense. I don't do that anymore. I've always been a long-term investor, not a stock trader. Making short-term bets on the market, that's just gambling. But, here's the thing: "long-term" takes on a new meaning when you're my age. When I had that Covid thing last year, I didn't know if I'd be around much longer. I still don't know. So, long-term isn't very long when you're 75. You can't plan for the future because... well, time is short. You can't plan anything, really, because you don't know how long you have to see it through.

> Time remaining
> 25 minutes

Jane        You feel paralyzed by the uncertainty.

> *A successful intervention often elicits further,*
> *previously unstated material, as it appears*
> *has happened here, but this example is*
> *given without recognition of its emotional*
> *content: frustration, anger, despair. So Jane*
> *returns to the Rogerian approach. A more*
> *helpful response might have been to note the*
> *lingering effects of his bout of serious illness*
> *("that Covid thing") on his current thinking.*
> *Jane knew about that recent illness from his*
> *history, but, so far, she has not factored it*
> *into her formulation.*

Charles     (Nodding) Exactly. Or here's another way of think-
            ing about it. It's like I'm in a small boat in the middle
            of a big river. There's no motor, not even a pair of
            oars. I'm being swept along by the current and ahead
            of me I can hear the falls and I know I'm going over
            them but I don't know how far ahead they are. Could
            be ten miles or one mile or 500 yards. I can't tell. But
            I know when I get there it's all over for me.

Jane        And you're not frightened, out there in that rudder-
            less boat?

*Charles uses his own metaphor but his*
*RHETORIC doesn't include an emotional*
*component. Jane's Rogerian response might*
*have been, "You feel helpless in the face of*
*an uncertain future" or "Like the boat you*
*have no control over your future." Jane*
*reacts, instead, to the missing emotional*
*component of his example.*

Charles    The fear is there but I'm trying to ignore it.

Jane    How's that working out for you?

*Again, she might have offered a restatement,*
*such as, "Acknowledging the fear makes it*
*more real," but the active response is too*
*tempting.*

Charles    (Chuckles) Not so well. Otherwise I wouldn't be sitting here.

Jane    I've been noticing something I want to point out to you.
You're talking about things that make you unhappy,
even fearful and... distraught, but your words and
your feelings don't match up. The end of your life is
approaching, you don't know when; yet as you discuss
it, it's like you're talking about your golf game.

*Jane decides to break from Rogerian*
*technique by a METACOMMUNICATION*
*that confronts Charles with the disparity*
*between his ideas and his emotions. When a*
*therapist who usually asks questions makes*
*a clear statement, the contrast often gives*
*the statement extra weight and impact. In*
*this case, however, she has been making*
*"Rogerian" statements with very few*
*questions, so the contrast may be negligible.*

| Charles | (Calmly, but with an edge to his voice) What do you expect me to do... wail and scream, rend my garments? Roll on the floor? It's not going to change anything. |
|---|---|

Jane        You don't think that mismatch is important? That you can talk about something as upsetting as death without feeling any emotion?

> *This slight show of anger is the most he has allowed so far. Jane sticks with her point. She sharpens the disparity, but uses the general, more intellectual and less challenging term "emotion" rather than naming specific feelings.*

Charles     Listen, that's just the way I am. The way I've always been. I keep my feelings in check and keep them to myself. It's called compartmentalizing. When I was working, you had to stay calm in the face of other people's distress. Otherwise, if both of you fell apart, nothing would ever be accomplished. You know the old saying, "if you can keep your head while all about you others are losing theirs..." So that's me. I'm good at keeping my head. I don't let my emotions take over.

Jane        Perhaps that's what's making it so hard for you to deal with this.

> *Jane makes the point directly for him, with the implied suggestion that he needs to change his behavior if he hopes to deal with the problem that brought him to see her. She notes that this defensive walling off of emotion is EGO SYNTONIC and wonders if the partial failure of his "compartmentalizing" that occurred when he began to ruminate over his approaching*

> *death occurred because his feelings*
> *overwhelmed him and, using his metaphor,*
> *"broke out of their compartment."*

Charles        (Tilts his head to the side) You could be right.

Jane           Compartmentalizing didn't work with your worries about dying.

> *She wants to undermine his satisfaction*
> *with his habit of walling off his feelings and*
> *perhaps allow him to let more of them come*
> *through.*

Charles        I hadn't thought of it that way.

Jane           So maybe it's useful in some circumstances, like in a business meeting, but not so good for personal issues. How did you develop that skill?

> *She declines to overtly NAME this defense as*
> *ISOLATION OF AFFECT. That might backfire if he*
> *just factors it into his intellectualized approach*
> *or it might help as another way to shift it to*
> *EGO DYSTONIC. Instead, she acknowledges*
> *compartmentalizing as a "skill" but hopes to*
> *show him it works against him when applied to*
> *his personal feelings. To build a FOUNDATION*
> *for this effort she asks him for more history.*

> Time remaining
> 15 minutes

Charles        Hmmm. I'm not sure. (Thinks a moment) Well, I guess I had to. I come from a very emotional family. My parents were always bickering with each other. My sister was what people call a drama queen. Our house was never a calm place.

| | |
|---|---|
| Jane | I don't remember you mentioning your sister. Was she older or younger than you? |

> *The emergence of new historical information sidetracks the planned discussion.*

| | |
|---|---|
| Charles | (Microexpression: distaste?) Cassandra. Three years younger. I don't see much of her these days. She lives clear across the country. She wanted to be an actress. (Grimaces) No surprise there! But that didn't work out so she had a career in the production side of the movies. She's retired now. Lives with her partner and a couple of cats. |

| | |
|---|---|
| Jane | Are you saying Cassandra is gay? |

> *Charles has avoided the label, another indication of his evading possible emotional topics.*

| | |
|---|---|
| Charles | I'm afraid so. |

| | |
|---|---|
| Jane | You don't approve of her? |

> *She tries to elicit his feelings about his sister. She might better have asked directly what were his feelings about her being gay.*

| | |
|---|---|
| Charles | (Shrugs) Not my place to approve or disapprove. Like I said, we're not close. |

| | |
|---|---|
| Jane | I don't know. First you called her a "drama queen." Then you said her career was a failure and now you imply that her choice of a partner was… regrettable. Doesn't that sound like you're not very proud of her? |

> *He says he has no feelings at all about her. Although he might have an opinion or a judgment about his sister and simply*

*not wish to air it, Jane suspects he has so successfully defended against unpleasant feelings that he is actually unaware of how he feels toward Cassandra.*

*She suggests another response—"not very proud"—and again it might have worked better to ask him to describe his attitude to his sister. If he continued to avoid any emotional response, Jane might then be able to confront him with his "compartmentalizing" even about a family member.*

Charles   She's not a factor in my life. Not my circus, not my monkeys.

Jane   But growing up in your family, wasn't that your circus then? If she was the drama queen in the family maybe you had to be the stoic one. What do you think?

*Jane picks up his metaphor and makes her point with it, a good use of DICTION. She may have too little FOUNDATION for this INTERPRETATION, however.*

Charles   (Stiffens) What I meant was that my family, growing up, was like living in a… I don't know what to call it. Maybe, like a soap opera. Everything was a crisis. Not only my sister but my parents couldn't agree on anything. It was always an argument about something.

Jane   So you mean you had to be the calm one? What, like a peacemaker?

*He explains as a way of deflecting her interpretation, a consequence of her inadequate FOUNDATION. She tries again.*

| | |
|---|---|
| Charles | No, I wasn't the peacemaker. I just tried to stay out of it. I was better off when I was at school and away from all that. |
| Jane | I see. And both your parents are gone now? |

*Having failed twice with her effort to have him focus on his role in the family, she moves on.*

| | |
|---|---|
| Charles | Yes. My father died, let's see, it's 28 years ago now, and my mother died four years later, so she's gone 24 years. |
| Jane | How old was he? |

*Trust an accountant to come up with the numbers, Jane thinks, noting that numbers don't carry the emotion of losing his parents. She asks for his age, thinking his father's death might have more relevance to his own worries than his mother's.*

| | |
|---|---|
| Charles | My father? He was 76. A year older than me now. |
| Jane | Does that figure into your worries? That you're almost the same age as he was when he died? |

*Jane has now moved completely away from the "client-centered" approach she had decided on and is taking an active exploratory role, although she is having no more success with it than with the Rogerian approach.*

| | |
|---|---|
| Charles | I think about that. |
| Jane | And what thoughts do you have? |

> *"Think," not feel. She accepts his term in the interest of gathering more history.*

Charles    He had heart troubles and he sort of went downhill over that last year until one day he didn't wake up. He had a lot of time to get used to the idea that he would die. I wonder how he coped with it.

Jane    "One day he just didn't wake up." Isn't that what you were thinking a little while ago, that you might "wake up dead?"

> *She is able to link his father's death with his own worry, a possible important* ANTECEDENT *of his current fear.*

Charles    (Looks startled) Hey, you're right.

Jane    So, did you ever discuss it with him? His declining health. His approaching death?

> *She expects the answer to be "no" but wants to get it "on the record."*

Charles    Not a chance. We all ignored it, pretended he was all right. It wasn't a topic for discussion.

Jane    So when it came to that topic, everybody was stoic about it?

> *She* REFRAMES *his response ("stoic") as a way to characterize his avoidance of affect with the intention of later suggesting that it is not the best way for him to handle his fears.*

Charles    As far as I know. I was, anyway. I didn't know what to say to him.

| | |
|---|---|
| Jane | Suppose you could talk to him about it now. What would you say? |

> *She introduces a new TACTIC, quasi-role-playing, a technique more common in the experiential therapies, in the hope that it will allow Charles to release some of the affect she assumes is bound up in his father's last illness and demise.*

| | |
|---|---|
| Charles | No idea. I wouldn't know how to start. It'd be different if he brought it up himself. |

| | |
|---|---|
| Jane | All right. Suppose I'm him, and I say to you, "You know, Charles, I'm dying of this heart problem." |

> *She tries again with a more explicit role-playing.*

| | |
|---|---|
| Charles | I guess I'd say, "I know you are and I'm sorry." |

Time remaining
5 minutes

| | |
|---|---|
| Jane | And then I might say, "So I hope you'll look out for your mother and your sister." |

> *Since Jane knows so little about his father, she has no basis for "quoting" him in this role-playing exercise. A better choice may have been to ask Charles what his father would say in response.*

| | |
|---|---|
| Charles | He wouldn't include my sister. He never could accept her being a lesbian. He never mentioned her after she started living with her partner. |

| | |
|---|---|
| Jane | Earlier, you said your family was like a soap opera, but it sounds like, in spite of all the uproar, some topics were off limits. Is that right? |

*Charles disrupts the role-playing as he contradicts her offered statement. Jane abandons the exercise and returns to her initial line of inquiry. She introduces a new NAME ("uproar") to suggest that the high emotional levels in the family were difficult for Charles.*

Charles    I hadn't thought about it that way, but I think you're right.

Jane    So would you say that compartmentalizing was a family trait?

*Charles again agrees with one of her ideas without much of an emotional component. It's as if they're having an intellectual chat and he acknowledges it when she makes a good point. One indication that this discussion is unproductive is that it has failed to elicit much additional or useful history. Jane tries another question. Her use of his earlier term, compartmentalizing, not only provides a link but also focuses the problem for future discussion. The six-syllable word (perhaps a management theory term) epitomizes the intellectualization and the emotional isolation inherent in his coping mechanism. Jane hopes that by emphasizing these qualities she can help him overcome them.*

Charles    You think my father did the same thing I do? Yeah, I guess he did.

Jane    As children we learn by imitating what the significant adults do.

*Jane responds with a statement. She offers
this NORMALIZING generalization as a way to
circumvent his resistance to being "just like
your father" and to elicit more childhood
evidence of it. A better approach might have
been to ask a direct question about how he is
like his father.*

Charles     That doesn't sound like a bad thing.

Jane        It's not bad in and of itself, but it could be a problem
            if it keeps someone from dealing with problems they
            might otherwise solve.

            *Now she is forced to continue with the
            generalization. This kind of discussion,
            general and impersonal, is unlikely to move
            the work forward.*

Charles     Like me and my worries about dying?

Jane        Don't you think that's true?

            *Fortunately, Charles makes it personal again.
            Jane tries to take advantage of his observation
            by asking for more of his thoughts about it.*

Charles     I don't know. It's not that I don't think about it. I
            think about it all the time. That's the opposite of com-
            partmentalizing, isn't it?

Jane        Not exactly. What you're compartmentalizing isn't
            the topic itself but your feelings about it. I think that's
            what keeping you from a resolution.

            *Charles is comfortable with this intellectual
            discussion. Jane is forced to continue with*

> *a further generalization, but she tries to*
> *bring it onto a personal level.*

Charles      I don't know about that. I think I have a lot of feelings about it. Dying, that is. I may not show it. I'm not someone who wears his heart on his sleeve.

Jane         We need to talk more about that, but our time is up for today and we have to stop.

> *All she can do now, since time has run out, is*
> *suggest they continue to discuss it.*

Charles      Sure.

### Discussion

Charles' intellectual style presents a challenge. On the one hand, he confronts an existential threat that has motivated him to seek therapy. On the other hand, he remains emotionally distant from it and acts as if it will yield to rational investigation. Charles' isolation from the feelings that such a serious threat should engender keeps him mired in his despair even as he intellectualizes about it.

Charles is the kind of patient who readily engages with the therapist, but may fail to make any significant progress in resolving his presenting problem. The absence of affective experiencing, a key element in the generation of helpful behavioral change, will undermine therapeutic progress. Charles' rationality is not likely to resolve his crisis. Jane's empathy with him in the absence of observable affect is, at best, useless and, at worst, counterproductive. Their work together could result in a long-term period of therapy without any significant benefit. Charles could remain in therapy with her until he dies, discussing his dilemma from behind his intellectual shield, without ever resolving the problem that brought him to treatment.

This first therapy session has been relatively unsuccessful. Jane's goal was "to help Charles overcome his current affective isolation."

His affective isolation is not merely "current" but it is a longstanding and entrenched defense. Nothing Jane tried seemed to make any dent in his intellectual shell, not her original effort to be **with** the patient, not discussing other people's ideas through their quotations, not directly confronting him on his restricted affect, his "compartmentalizing." Her various strategies—client-centered, CBT, interpretations, even role-playing—all failed to advance the work. Jane might be justified in thinking that Charles' defensive armor will leave him unreceptive to her efforts. Through all the frustrations of the session, however, the therapeutic alliance remained intact, a positive factor that could still lead to a satisfactory outcome. Jane needs to reexamine her treatment plan, especially with regard to what therapeutic modality will be most helpful.

## SESSION THREE

Today, Charles wears an open-neck dress shirt and dark slacks. His hair is uncombed. He arrives just in time for his appointment. He looks tense and uncomfortable as he takes his seat.

Time remaining
45 minutes

Charles       Sorry I'm late. I had to rush over here. We've had a death in the family.

Jane          Oh?

*Jane notes that he's not actually late. Just not as early as before. Not sure what he's talking about, she uses the minimal questioning response, waiting to hear more. She observes how less formally he is dressed today, perhaps a clue to his mental state and an indication they may be able to make more progress than before, depending on whatever the source of his distress turns out to be.*

| | |
|---|---|
| Charles | (Grimaces) Betsy, our Miniature Schnauzer died. Completely unexpected. Found her this morning when I came down for breakfast. |
| Jane | Quite a shock. |
| | *Not what she expected to hear. She responds with a* METACOMMUNICATIVE *statement while waiting to see where this will go.* |
| Charles | Yes. We had her since she was a puppy. We were all very attached to her. |
| Jane | Attached? |
| | *She flags the intellectual word he uses instead of a more emotional term; for example, "loved."* |
| Charles | She was part of our family for 14 years. |
| Jane | I see. |
| | *Jane is uncertain how this event will fit into therapy, especially whether Charles will deal with his emotional response to the loss.* |
| Charles | (Rubbing his forehead with his fingertips) Now I'll probably never have another Schnauzer. |
| Jane | Never? |
| | *Jane picks up on his all-or-nothing response (a CBT flag), behind which may lie his primary fear of dying.* |
| Charles | Yeah. I couldn't take on the responsibility. I don't know if I'll be around long enough. (He sighs) |
| Jane | You're afraid a new pet might outlive you? |

> *She restates his assertion with the more emotional word, "afraid," as the focus, a NAMING TACTIC.*

Charles   That's right. When you bring a dog into your family you have to be responsible for them. Housebreaking. Obedience training. Then they're dependent on you and you have to be there for them.

Jane   So, just like having a new child.

> *Another restatement with an INTERPRETATION that he means any "family" member.*

Charles   (Nods. He looks teary-eyed. He brings out a handkerchief and wipes his eyes, then blows his nose.)

Jane   I can see this loss has really upset you.

> *She wants him to focus on his feelings rather than the intellectual side of this death. This METACOMMUNICATION brings their attention onto his emotional state rather than the words he is using.*

Charles   (Sniffles) It does.

Jane   Can you put how you feel into words?

> *Jane tries a direct invitation. She toys with the idea of pointing out that Betsy "woke up dead," exactly the fear to which Charles alluded in the previous session, but she decides it would sound insensitive used here.*

Charles   (Shakes his head. A few tears roll down his cheek.) I don't know.

Jane   Just say what you're feeling.

> *This instructive invitation shows Jane is feeling frustrated by his lack of response. A better tactic would have been to remain silent.*

Charles    (Stares at the floor) It's a big loss. Makes me wonder how my family is going to feel when I go.

Jane    Uh-huh.

> *He can't reach the emotional dimension of this loss but at least he sees its relevance to his existential problem. Jane makes a neutral comment that invites further discussion.*

Charles    What if it was me? What if my wife woke up tomorrow and found me next to her. Dead.

Jane    Do you have any health problems that would lead to your sudden and unexpected passing?

> *She knows he doesn't. Her FOUNDATIONAL question is a CBT intervention: confronting him with his NEGATIVE OVERGENERALIZATION. This TACTIC is not helpful in this context, however, and might divert him away from the more important topic. More to the point might be: "How would your wife react" or even "What would she do." It is a minor misjudgment but nevertheless a missed opportunity.*

Charles    Not that I know of, no. But that doesn't mean it couldn't happen. When I was so sick with the virus last year I didn't know if I'd make it or not. If I had to go into the hospital I might have never come out. (Pauses) I feel much older than I did before my illness.

Jane         Do you think that's when you started to focus on your mortality? When you felt you had had a close call?

*Charles brings up an important new aspect, that his serious illness is what provoked this crisis. Jane had missed the importance of this experience before, so this idea is kind of an "Aha" moment for her. (If she wasn't sitting in front of the client, she might have struck her forehead with the heel of her hand and muttered, "Dummy!") She realizes she now must revise her FORMULATION to include both the existential and situational categories; namely, that a life-threatening illness provoked an EXISTENTIAL CRISIS, overwhelming his intellectual defenses.*

Charles      Probably. I mean, I'd thought about it before, but then it looked like I might not be around, and I started to think about what would happen afterwards.

                                                        Time remaining
                                                        35 minutes

Jane         Like what?

*"Probably" is his way of not fully acknowledging any worrying thought. She wants to hear as much about this new connection as possible and invites him to elaborate. Meanwhile, Jane is mulling over how best to use her now revised FORMULATION.*

Charles      Like... books that would be published that I'd never read, sports teams that I follow and I wouldn't see the next season. My grandchildren growing up. My wife would be all alone. (He breathes a big sigh and shakes his head) You know, animals don't have this kind of worry. They live in the present moment. Betsy lived in the present. She didn't think about her death. Dogs don't worry about dying. It's only us humans that look ahead. We can't know how long we have, but we know that it's coming. For all our science and technology we're helpless when it comes to ourselves.

Jane   It's the uncertainty about the future? Is that the hardest part for you?

> *His sudden change of subject to the abstract idea of animals' consciousness suggests he wants to avoid thinking about the effect his death might have on the people he loves. Jane misses an opportunity here. She picks up the abstract concept rather than the distress at his family's loss.*

Charles   I'd be better off if I lived in the moment like Betsy. It's the not knowing.

Jane   Is that the core of this? That it's out of your control?

> *Jane RENAMES "not knowing" as "no control." She attempts to focus on one aspect of his personality that increases his struggle with the concept of dying.*

Charles   I suppose it is. Sounds ridiculous, doesn't it? But recognizing that doesn't make it any easier.

Jane   What if you knew the answer. What if you knew that you'd die exactly one year from today? Would that make things easier for you?

> *He brushes it off with his comment that it makes no difference, perhaps suggesting it's not a problem after all.*

*She tries an indirect approach, rather than confronting him on his rejection of the "control" idea. Meanwhile, she has yet to focus on the impact of his Covid-19 illness.*

Charles   (Jerks back) That would be worse!

Jane   Worse?

*At last a true emotional moment. Jane flags it with a one-word reference.*

Charles   You bet. I'm already paralyzed by the thought I could go at any time and nothing I can do will change that. If I knew when… well, it would leave me completely incapacitated. I mean, what would be the point of doing anything? That's how I feel anyway.

Jane   So, then, you wouldn't continue what you're doing now? No more fundraising? The animal shelter? Being a volunteer?

*He uses "feel" when he means "think," since he hasn't expressed his feelings in any direct way. She challenges his OVERGENERALIZATION.*

Charles   There'd be no point.

Jane   I want to go back to something you said a few moments ago, about your wife and your grandchildren. How do you feel when you think about them after your death?

*Realizing how far off the track the discussion has gone, Jane interrupts to redirect it to the point she missed earlier.*

Charles   I don't know.

Jane        You don't know? That thought seemed to upset you.
            Can you say more about that?

            *She uses the general term, "upset," to avoid*
            *suggesting what his emotional response*
            *"should" be.*

Charles     (Stares at his hands for several seconds. He seems to
            be trying to hold back his emotions.)

Jane        What are you feeling now?

            *Continuing to urge him like this may become*
            *counterproductive. He may resent her pressure*
            *rather than focusing on his inner response.*

Charles     (Big sigh) I guess that is the hardest part for me.
            Leaving them all behind. Not knowing how their
            lives will go on without me. (Shakes his head) It's
            stupid, really. What difference will it make? I'll
            never know.

Jane        That sounds like how you're thinking about it, not
            how you're feeling about it. What about the emotional
            response to these thoughts?

            *He seems to contain his feelings, perhaps*
            *in reaction to Jane's question. A better*
            *response here might have been for her to*
            *remain silent. Jane continues to prod him.*

Charles     I don't know. Maybe that's more than I can handle.
            I'm already feeling too much.

Jane        You're afraid you'd be overwhelmed? That you
            wouldn't be able to handle the emotional side of this
            problem?

            *"Already feeling too much" may be an*
            *indirect message to Jane, meaning "leave*

*me alone." She tries to recover by restating his thought.*

Charles     (Charles remains quiet for a few moments, staring at his hands held in his lap) You quoted something from Hamlet at our meeting last week and I went back and read the play again and, at the end, when he's facing the possibility that his uncle plans to kill him, he says something like—and I can't quote it exactly—he says if I don't die now I will later, and if it's not later it'll be now, but whether it's now or later it **will** still happen. And then he says—and this is what stuck with me—he says, "the readiness is all." And that's it, isn't it? The readiness.

Jane     (Nodding) Today we might call it acceptance.

*Jane RENAMES Hamlet's word with its modern equivalent. She wants to reinforce Charles' recognition of this idea, intellectualized though it may be. It is, after all, the outcome of her work with him that she felt would be most helpful, the AIM at the top of her treatment plan. Once she constructs a new formulation, based on her recognition of the precipitating event— Charles' bout with Covid—she may need to reexamine and update the treatment plan.*

Charles     I guess I'm not there yet. Why is it so hard for me?

Jane     Any ideas?

*She declines to provide her thoughts and asks him to do more work on his own.*

Charles     I don't know. In a way it's ridiculous. I could have another 20 years yet and I'm stuck with thinking it's going to be tomorrow. Maybe I'm making myself crazy for no reason.

Time remaining<br>25 minutes

Jane    Yes, but doesn't "readiness" or acceptance mean you're prepared for it if it does happen tomorrow?

*He backs away from the new concept. She tries to keep him on it.*

Charles    That's not acceptance. That's... what's the word? That's resignation. It's giving up without a fight.

Jane    Giving up what? Fighting who?

*She challenges the intellectual abstractions.*

Charles    (Shakes his head) I don't know. Fate, I guess. I wish I could just stop thinking about this and live day to day.

Jane    You said something earlier that might be important for us to look into, that this all started when you were ill with Covid and you thought you might not survive it.

*Jane belatedly returns to her earlier recognition that his life-threatening illness is an important determinant of his present distress. It also provides something concrete and real on which to focus the discussion, rather than the abstract "existential threat."*

Charles    I hadn't thought about that lately. Maybe you're right. I'll think about it.

Jane    Can you say a little more about your experience with the virus? How did it start? How long were you ill?

*"I'll think about it" means "but not now."*
*His attempt to put it off suggests it may be an*
*important piece of the problem. She ignores*
*his deflection and asks for details rather than*
*let the discussion focus on an abstraction.*

Charles          (Frowns) It started on a weekend. Saturday morning I
                 thought I was coming down with a cold. My nose was
                 running and then I realized I wasn't smelling things.
                 My sense of smell was just gone and the food tasted
                 funny too. By the end of the day I was feeling hot
                 and achy and I had a fever of 104. I went to bed that
                 night but I had trouble sleeping because I felt so sick
                 and the next morning I stayed in bed. I was cough-
                 ing and I just wanted to sleep. So I still wasn't sure
                 it was Covid. I had just got the first vaccine dose the
                 week before, but I guess the virus was already in me.
                 I don't know. (He pauses, staring at his hands)

Jane             Then what happened?

                 *Her continuing interest emphasizes to*
                 *him the possible importance of this line of*
                 *inquiry.*

Charles          (Looks up) Well, it was the weekend so I didn't know
                 who to see about it. I didn't want to go to the emergency
                 room. I figured that would be a zoo. I might be there
                 for hours and I didn't feel up to it. So I just waited it
                 out and by the next morning I was feeling a little bet-
                 ter. My fever was down. I stayed in bed all day and just
                 had some soup. But then it got worse again and I had
                 another bad night, so the next day I called the doctor's
                 office, but my doctor was out sick himself and they told
                 me to stay at home and rest, drink fluids, and they'd see
                 me if it got worse. Worse! I was already feeling worse.

| | |
|---|---|
| Jane | They didn't want you to come in and be seen? |
| | *She picks up on the one element that promises to evoke more emotion, his perception that his health care providers didn't care about him.* |
| Charles | No. Not unless I had trouble breathing or I turned blue. |
| Jane | That must have been scary. |
| | *She suggests a response, using a* METACOMMUNICATION, *instead of asking him to describe how he'd actually felt, which might have been the more helpful question.* |
| Charles | Yeah. Well, actually, I was more angry than scared. I mean, I get it now. Their office was probably overwhelmed with cases. Or maybe they were worried I was too contagious and would spread the virus around. I don't know. But at the time I felt neglected. Like they didn't care. I mean, by that time I realized it was this virus people were dying from and my doctor's office wasn't interested. |
| Jane | You were on your own. |
| | *Charles chooses to correct her about how he felt and to supply more about his reaction. Her response is a Rogerian restatement.* |
| Charles | Yeah. Fortunately my wife was there to take care of me and she didn't get sick. She'd got the vaccine a few weeks before I did so I guess she was protected. I put it off. Too busy or I didn't think it mattered or something. It was stupid of me. I could have died. |
| Jane | Was that on your mind at the time? |
| | *She asks whether his present fears are linked to the emotional events from the past.* |

| Charles | No. Only later. At the time I was too sick to worry about that. That sounds crazy, doesn't it? |

Time remaining<br>15 minutes

| Jane | Maybe the illness hit you like you were Betsy. You were only living in the present. |

> *Jane begins to* LAY A FOUNDATION *she hopes will let her use Betsy's death as a helpful metaphor for Charles.*

| Charles | Hah! You're right. I just wanted to get through the next hour. |

| Jane | So when did you start to worry about dying? How long after you recovered? |

> *She is still unclear about the link between his Covid illness and his current fear.*

| Charles | Not for some time. After the symptoms went away I felt okay. I didn't have that long-Covid thing people talk about. I was just glad I was over it. |

| Jane | So is what you're feeling now a kind of delayed reaction? You think it all goes back to when you were so sick? |

> *She asks again to clarify the link between his illness and his present fear of dying, although Charles has already made it pretty clear.*

| Charles | That sounds right. |

| Jane | Is there more to it? |

> *His answer seems more designed to agree for the sake of agreement, suggesting*

*that there may be other ANTECEDENTS as
important or more important.*

Charles    (Bends his head to stare at the floor) Maybe. I mean, after I recovered I was relieved. Glad to be alive, as they say. I didn't start to think about how I was still going to die until later.

Jane       Any idea what triggered that worry to start?

           *Jane pursues the missing ANTECEDENT.*

Charles    (Looks up at her) Actually, I do. I read that some- one important at my college had died. My alumni magazine came and he was on the cover. Turns out he was a big star in their endowment program. He'd made them tons of money. The magazine was full of tributes to him. He was a great guy, a great friend, a financial genius, and on and on. And I thought, so what? All that success and now he's dead and every- thing he achieved is meaningless. And then I started thinking about myself the same way.

Jane       How so?

           *Now that Jane seems to be on the right
           track, Charles produces some new, possibly
           significant history. Recognizing the importance
           of this event, Jane asks for more detail.*

Charles    (Sits up straight, looking at Jane) He was younger than me when he died. The magazine gave him a big spread. People wrote about him, how he helped them become better, how he was such an inspiring teacher, he was a help to others. Encomiums from students, fellow faculty people. You'd think he was the best thing to ever happen to them. And so what? (His voice rises) So fucking what! Now he's dead and all that good stuff doesn't mean a thing to him. He's rotting in his grave. Like I told you before, that thing from Tolstoy: what meaning has life that death does not destroy.

Jane    (After waiting to see if he'll continue) And you see the same fate for yourself? That after you're gone, whatever effect you had on the people around you won't matter? I mean, won't it still matter to them?

> *Jane begins a CBT approach by examining the premise Charles implies in this comparison of himself and the man who was so important to his college. That premise seems to be: your life doesn't matter unless you're around to experience it. She starts by making the comparison explicit.*

Charles    But I won't be alive to appreciate it.

Jane    Then I suppose you feel that any satisfactions you get in life have to be appreciated while you're still alive. Isn't that right?

> *She introduces the new premise in the form of a question.*

Charles    (Shrugs) Sure.

Jane    Well, here's a thought experiment. Suppose Betsy could read and she saw that quote from Tolstoy. Would she give up on her life or would she say, I've got today so let me get the most out of it that I can?

> *She uses this "Betsy" metaphor to suggest an alternative to his premise. The RHETORIC allows her to present a different point of*

*view without the disapproval Charles might feel (and reject out of hand) if she used him as the example. His positive feelings for his pet and companion make Betsy an agreeable example, one he is more likely to accept.*

Charles        (Laughs) The question answers itself.

Time remaining
5 minutes

Jane        It does, doesn't it?

*Her TACTIC is successful. He can buy into the new concept without having to defend himself as having had the "wrong" idea.*

Charles        Betsy was always a happy dog.

Jane        Uh-huh.

*She acknowledges his agreement in order to bolster his shift in point of view.*

Charles        If Betsy were here she'd probably tell me that I'm spoiling today by worrying about tomorrow.

Jane        Smart dog!

*He applies it to himself without her having to make it as a prescription he must follow. She wants to encourage him to use this idea to help himself.*

Charles        Yes. (Pauses to think it through) That's helpful.

Jane        Good.

*More reinforcement.*

Charles   One of Betsy's puppies, she's full grown now, just had a litter. They're not purebred. Just some male dog she encountered along the way. So a mixed breed. And the owner called me to see if I knew how she can get them into good homes. Now I'm thinking I might take one of them myself. It wouldn't be Betsy, but I'd like to have a remembrance of her.

Jane   A new start.

*Charles has reversed his earlier position that he would not be able to take the responsibility for a new dog because he might die and not be around to take care of it. This spontaneous plan suggests that the preceding therapeutic work has made an important change in his approach to his view of this new stage of his life. Whether it persists and helps him approach his end remains to be seen, and will no doubt require further working through in future sessions.*

Charles   Yes.

Jane   Our time is up and we have to stop. See you next week.

*Jane declines to continue the discussion, important as it may be, in order to maintain the session boundaries. She implies that they can make as much progress in the next session as they might if she prolonged this one.*

Charles   Sure.

### Discussion

This second therapy session was important for two new developments in the evolution of Charles' treatment.

The first was the way an exogenous event—in this case the unexpected death of Betsy, a beloved family pet—offered an unusual opportunity to break through the intellectual defenses Charles had been using, with only limited success, to shield himself from his ruminations on his own mortality. One "benefit" of this development was that they were no longer discussing an abstraction, and a future abstraction, at that; namely, that Charles would no longer exist at some point at an unknown time. In effect, Charles was grieving a loss that he had not yet suffered and that, when it occurred, he would no longer be there to experience it. (If she had selected a different therapy approach than her client-centered strategy Jane might have usefully employed this idea.)

Instead, the death of the family dog was an immediate, concrete event with a real "member of the family." Charles was able to overcome his intellectual defenses and express his grief more openly, including shedding a few tears during the session. Charles also recalled that, prior to the session, he was already beginning to modify his outlook. His response to Hamlet's acceptance ("The readiness is all") shows that he had taken over the idea for himself. The discussion of Betsy's presumed approach to life, that she lived in the moment and didn't worry about her future demise, allowed Charles to consider the same attitude. One could almost say that Charles used partial identifications with both Hamlet and Betsy to facilitate his acceptance of this idea. This healthier approach is not yet fully realized and integrated. It will require further therapeutic work in future sessions. In any event, Charles' decision to adopt one of Betsy's puppies is a hopeful development and perhaps a sign that the therapy will have a positive outcome.

The second development was Jane's belated recognition, well into the second session, that Charles' encounter with a Covid infection was the immediate, initial cause of his preoccupation with his own death. The harsh realities of the epidemic represented an actual existential threat: over a million dead, the specter of protracted disability from "long-Covid," the danger of unwitting contact with infected people, the disrupted social structure with its impact on families, on commerce, on friendships, the unseen menace in the air. Jane must review for herself how she overlooked such an obvious dynamic, central to Charles' whole presentation. Perhaps she will find that her own reluctance to confront the realities of illness and death created this blind spot.

What felt to Charles like a near-death experience had broken through his denial of a possibly approaching end. He could no longer ignore it. Jane had missed an obvious and important antecedent and needed to adjust her formulation to it. Although Jane was unable to pivot in mid-session to reformulate and modify her treatment plan, her recognition of the importance of Charles' experience with Covid will undoubtedly improve her subsequent work with him. As discussed in the chapter "General Principles of Psychotherapy", as the formulation evolves through the accumulation of new and more accurate information, the treatment plan must be modified to reflect these changes, and the revised formulations will, hopefully, be successive approximations of the truth.

The crushing existential weight of a person's recognition that life will end is a difficult topic for both patient and therapist. Jane struggled with it and had difficulty maintaining a consistent therapeutic strategy.

## Notes

1 See the chapter "General Principles of Psychotherapy."
2 Andrew Marvell, "To His Coy Mistress," 1681.
3 Originally credited to Samuel Johnson ("Depend upon it, Sir, when a man knows he is to be hanged in a fortnight, it concentrates the mind wonderfully") but also to Mark Twain: "nothing so focuses the mind as the prospect of being hanged."
4 Leo Tolstoy, *A Confession*, 1882.
5 "Why, then, 'tis none to you, for there is nothing either good or bad, but thinking makes it so." Hamlet II:2,247–249.

## Reference

Rogers, C. R. (1965). *Client-Centered Therapy*. Houghton Mifflin.

# Sophie

## A Discouraged Divorcée

### Referral

Sophie is a 46 year old private patient. She consulted her gynecologist because of lack of energy, loss of interest in her usual activities and poor sleep, which Sophie attributed to going through menopause. She gave Sophie a prescription for Xanax (alprazolam) and referred her to Jane with a diagnosis of "depression."

### History

Jane saw Sophie for an initial interview. She said her problem was, "I don't know what to do. My future looks blank."

Sophie and her husband, Dontrell, married when she was 25 and he was 30, They have two children: Alicia, age 20, who manages one of her father's restaurants, and Jamal, 17, who is a senior in high school. Four years earlier, Dontrell announced he wanted a divorce. He is the owner of three MacDonald's franchises and Sophie knew he had had extramarital relationships with several of his employees. She learned that he now wanted to marry one of them. The divorce proceedings dragged on for eight months during which Dontrell, having moved out, lived in an apartment with his new girlfriend, Kinesha. During these eight months Sophie was distracted and had a poor appetite. She lost 11 pounds. She has now gained back the weight but not her interest in food. In the divorce settlement, Sophie received full ownership of their house and a monthly alimony payment, along with child support for Jamal until he reaches age 18.

DOI: 10.4324/9781003353003-8

Sophie is the oldest child and only daughter from an intact family. Her father was a driver for UPS who is now retired, and her mother, who stayed at home to raise the children, now works at the local supermarket. One brother drives for UPS and the other is in the Army. Sophie graduated high school and found a job with a large insurance company. She stopped working when she became pregnant with Alicia. Sophie has no close friends or social groups. Her isolation has increased as both Dontrell and Alicia have left the home and Jamal has one foot out the door. Jane wonders if she came not for therapy, but just to have someone to talk to. Sophie's motivation for change was moderate, but her motivation for therapy was weak, saying "I don't know what good it could do."

## Mental Status Examination

Sophie was an alert, pleasant-appearing, heavyset woman dressed in a long-sleeved black sweater over blue slacks. She was mildly agitated and restless in the interview, occasionally wringing her hands and nervously smoothing her hair. Her speech was soft and somewhat fretful. Her mood was diffusely unhappy but not depressed. She denied feelings of hopelessness and suicidal thoughts, but said she felt "blah" most of the time and had no energy to do housework or other routine activities. She described her menopause experience as "I'm not even a woman anymore." She reported having wine with dinner and often had a "nightcap" to help her fall asleep.

## Formulation

Jane was puzzled after the initial interview about how to understand Sophie's present difficulties. She did not meet criteria for major depression and her clinical presentation seemed to be more pervasive than an adjustment disorder. Instead of these more formal diagnoses, Jane concluded that Sophie is failing to make a life transition. Her marriage has ended, one child has left the home and the second will be gone soon, while her menopausal experience has left her feeling uncertain of even her biological status. Her identity components as a wife, a mother and a woman have all been challenged by the changes in her life circumstances.

(Formulation Category: Developmental)

## Treatment Plan

Based on this analysis, Jane contemplated a therapy AIM along the lines of consolidating a new self-identity. Possible GOALS to help her achieve this transition include coming to terms with her grown children leaving, reexamining her life ambitions, both socially and in regard to work, and in general moving on with life after her divorce. While these objectives seem somewhat vague, they nevertheless provide a way forward for the therapy. Jane expects that a combination of directive and existential therapies will be needed.

Jane explains her idea to Sophie and suggests they meet for six more sessions to see if they can make progress. If not, they can reevaluate whether therapy is worth continuing. Sophie suggests they might know enough after three sessions and Jane accepts this modification in order to reach a TREATMENT CONTRACT.

## SESSION TWO

Sophie arrives a few minutes early and sits slumped in the waiting room. She is again dressed in the black sweater and blue slacks. Her face shows no apparent makeup and her unwashed dark hair is mixed with gray. She walks slowly into Jane's office and slumps into a chair. She holds her handbag in her lap.

Time remaining
45 minutes

Jane        It's good to see you this morning.

*Jane senses her THERAPEUTIC ALLIANCE
with Sophie is weak and so she begins with
a friendly welcome. She notes that her
handbag is held in a defensive position.*

| | |
|---|---|
| Sophie | (Without making eye contact) Thank you. |
| Jane | Anything you want to tell me about since I last saw you? |

> *Again, Jane breaks her usual policy of discouraging a* CHRONICLE *as she tries to make a stronger connection with this client.*

| | |
|---|---|
| Sophie | (Sighs) Not really. (She falls silent as Jane waits) I had to call Dontrell because my alimony check was late. He said it was in the mail. |
| Jane | "Your check is in the mail." One of the three great lies. |

> *Jane wants to strengthen the* ALLIANCE *with this semi-humorous supportive remark.*

| | |
|---|---|
| Sophie | (Looks up) What are the other two? |
| Jane | "I'll respect you in the morning" is one and the other is "I'm from the government and I'm here to help you." |

> *She completes the witticism hoping that a shared chuckle might establish a better connection.*

| | |
|---|---|
| Sophie | (Smiles) |
| Jane | How often do you have to deal with Dontrell? |

> *Since Sophie brought up a problem with the ex-husband, Jane chooses this opening as a place to start exploring more of Sophie's challenges. "Start where the patient is at" is an old psychotherapy maxim but nevertheless valid.*

| | |
|---|---|
| Sophie | (Shakes her head) Not very often. He's usually pretty good with the check. And I might see him when he |

comes to pick up Jamal. He gets Jamal every other weekend.

Jane        How do you feel toward Dontrell?

*Now that she has a focus she wants to elicit more detail about their post-divorce relationship.*

Sophie      (After a silence) I don't feel anything. He's out of my life. It's over. He's gone his own way.

Jane        You're not angry?

*Jane thinks that anger is the missing component of Sophie's state of mind. She's not angry about the divorce, about the children leaving, about the changes in her body, or anything else. Her passive resignation is manifested in the diffuse sadness that has been mistaken for "depression." She takes the unusual step of suggesting an emotion because she senses that Sophie is not going to understand her feelings without help.*

Sophie      I was, back when it first happened. I'm not anymore.

Jane        When did the anger disappear?

*She wants to explore this change to see if it represents a healthy acceptance or the damaging suppression of a justified feeling.*

Sophie      (Looks around the room, as if searching for an answer) I don't know. I think it just faded away. The marriage was over. There was nothing I could do.

| Jane | You mean, you couldn't get him back? Did you want to? |

*Jane lightly challenges her apparent
acceptance of the divorce to see if it
provokes any emotion.*

| Sophie | Sometimes. When I was feeling lonely and I thought it would be nice to have somebody else around. |

| Jane | That doesn't sound like you had very strong feelings for him. If he was just a warm body to have around... Did your feelings for him change before the divorce? |

*Her current emotional presentation, to the
extent that it is a response to the divorce,
seems out of proportion. Her mood suggests
she was profoundly affected, but her
reported feelings are too mild to match. Jane
wonders if something else is bothering her
more, that she needs a different HYPOTHESIS.*

| Sophie | (Sighs) I guess they did. It wasn't a great marriage. By the end we were just living side by side. We barely spoke. |

Time remaining
35 minutes

| Jane | Are you saying it just fizzled out? You lost interest in him as he was drawing away from you? |

*Jane is still puzzled and again challenges
Sophie's apparent indifference. Her
persistence in doubting Sophie's reaction
reflects her difficulty giving up her
HYPOTHESIS about the "missing anger."*

| Sophie | (Sits up straighter) No. I wasn't losing interest. I was making a home. Cooking the meals, keeping the place clean, doing the shopping. Then, Alicia moved out. |

Jane                How did that change things?

> *Sophie is saying, past tense, that she had a stronger identity. This statement confirms an important component of Jane's FORMULATION. She could begin to explore that idea more but she chooses to continue with the history of the marriage. It could be a missed opportunity, but it is likely to come up again.*

Sophie              (Places her handbag on the floor) I'm not sure. She was working for Dontrell, so he still saw her, but I didn't. And then Dontrell started up with that woman. She was another one of his managers.

Jane                Are they still together? Dontrell and that woman?

> *Jane takes the removal of her handbag from her lap as a sign that Sophie is more relaxed. The fact that Alicia stopped seeing her mother seems significant but, again, it's a different topic. Jane stores it away with the intention of coming back to it later. For now, she continues to explore the relationship with Dontrell.*

Sophie              (Flatly) No idea.

Jane                You don't care?

> *Jane thinks Sophie does care but challenges her statement with a METACOMMUNICATION in the form of a question, where she has more chance of eliciting Sophie's true feelings.*

Sophie              (Irritated) Why should I? It's his life. He can do what he wants.

Jane                Okay. Now you sound kind of angry.

*She gets a response that seems to confirm her*
*HYPOTHESIS that Sophie is suppressing her anger*
*about the divorce and wants to confirm it using*
*another METACOMMUNICATION. The anger, in*
*the form of irritation, seems to be about Jane's*
*question. Jane's dedication to her HYPOTHESIS,*
*however, causes her to miss this nuance.*

Sophie        Yeah? Why, shouldn't I be?

Jane          Yes. Why shouldn't you be angry?

*Jane's repetition of Sophie's question serves*
*to support Sophie's recognition of her anger,*
*but, again, she doesn't connect it with her*
*questioning. Jane is focused on anger at*
*Dontrell while Sophie is irritated by Jane's*
*persistent interest in him. This divergence*
*weakens the THERAPEUTIC ALLIANCE.*

Sophie        So you think I should?

Jane          I'm surprised that you're not.

*Instead of keeping the focus on Sophie,*
*Jane elects to answer her question with a*
*statement of support. She still feels the need*
*to strengthen the THERAPEUTIC ALLIANCE and*
*sacrifices her neutral stance to that end.*

Sophie        (Shrugs) You can't stay angry forever.

Jane          You can still be angry and try not to think about it.
              If it's still there and you don't know it, that might do
              some damage.

*Sophie denies the emotion she just admitted*
*to. Jane still thinks it's about Dontrell. She*

*might have made an interpretative remark in the form of a question, such as "Does being angry make you uncomfortable?" but she has too little evidence at this early stage of therapy to support it, even in as tentative a form as a question. Instead, she settles for a NORMATIVE statement.*

Sophie      (Frowns) You think I'm damaged?

Jane        What do you think?

*This time she declines to give her opinion and turns the question back to Sophie. If she were to answer that, yes, she thinks Sophie might be "damaged," the THERAPEUTIC ALLIANCE would likely suffer.*

Sophie      (Stares at her hands, folded in her lap) Maybe I am. (She pauses and from her expression Jane thinks she may be about to bring up another topic. But then she shuts down and returns to Jane's question.) It's sure not the way I saw myself. Rattling around in the house with no family except for Jamal who's out more than he's home. I feel like a fat, stupid piece of junk nobody needs anymore. Might as well just throw me out. Like Dontrell. Found somebody new and a new place to live. (Pauses) I don't know what I'm doing. I don't know what I'm doing here.

Time remaining
25 minutes

Jane        I thought we agreed. What we're doing here is working on a way forward for you. You feel like you're stuck in the here and now. Nowhere to go and nothing to do. No wonder you no longer know who you are.

> *Of the various self-critical statements Sophie has listed, Jane chooses to respond to her expression of doubt about the therapy. If anything worthwhile is going to come from their work together, Sophie has to continue to attend. Jane's final sentence restates her HYPOTHESIS that Sophie's problem stems from a softening of her self-defined identity. Without using the actual term, identity, she attempts to RENAME Sophie's problem.*

Sophie    (Frowns) I know who I am. I just don't like the person I've become.

Jane    "The person you've become?" That's not the way it sounds to me. You're not a different person. You're still the old you: the mother, the wife, the homemaker. It's not you that changed. You're still the mother to Alicia and Jamal. You still see yourself as a wife. You still take care of the home. Isn't the problem that while you're the same, the things around you have changed? The kids are grown up. The husband left. The house no longer needs to be made into the family home. The old you is trying to do the things she always did, but those things are no longer there. They don't need the old you. You need a new you.

> *Jane restates the treatment plan in stronger terms. She not only challenges the self-pitying self-portrait Sophie painted but suggests she can become someone she would consider meaningful. She is able to state the central issue as a question with her declarative sentences simply as evidence.*

Sophie          (Skeptically) A new me? Who am I supposed to be
                now?

Jane            Well, that's up to you, isn't it? The first step might be
                you deciding what's next for you and how you can
                get there.

> *Sophie asks Jane for the answer. Jane spells
> it out in terms that give the choice to Sophie.
> The alternative—making suggestions as to
> what Sophie might do with her life now—
> would risk playing the transactional game,
> "why don't you yes but."[1]*

Sophie          (Querulous) But I had what I wanted. Those things
                you said. Then they all went away. Why do I have
                to find something new? Why is it up to me? It's not
                fair.

Jane            Are you thinking about the divorce?

> *Jane still thinks there is something more to the
> divorce than Sophie has so far revealed. In
> fact, she has a general sense that what Sophie
> has been willing to say is not the whole story.
> Since she has no evidence for this missing
> element, she does not confront Sophie with it.*

Sophie          Well, that's most of it. That's what started all this.

Jane            Dontrell started it.

> *Jane uses his name not only to keep the focus
> on Dontrell as the cause of Sophie's mood
> but also to encourage her to express the
> "missing" anger at the identified object.*

Sophie          That's right.

Jane          Any ideas about what made him do it?

              *She tries again.*

Sophie        (Nods her head) We just grew apart.

Jane          You know, that's not much of an explanation: "we
              just grew apart." Let's dig into that a little more.
              When did it start? What started it growing apart?
              Who grew apart first? Was it one thing or a bunch of
              things? You were married over 20 years. Were you
              growing apart all that time?

              > *Jane is reluctant to accept the idea that
              > Dontrell is not the source of the problem
              > for Sophie. But "digging in" to a topic
              > that Sophie may not care about carries
              > a risk. Her dogged pursuit may actually
              > damage the* THERAPEUTIC ALLIANCE *if Sophie
              > comes to feel that Jane does not understand
              > her.*

Sophie        I don't know. It's hard to say when it started. (Stares
              ahead for a moment) Well, I'll tell you where it
              started for me. It was when Alicia graduated high
              school. That was three years ago. We didn't know
              if she really would graduate. As soon as she turned
              14, she turned into a party girl. She was using drugs,
              getting high, there were a lot of boys. And not the
              nice kind. (Grimaces) So, she took up a lot of our
              time, trying to straighten her out, worrying about her.
              Then, at the end, she kind of pulled herself together
              and finally she graduated. Then Dontrell gave her a
              job at one of his stores and she's doing okay there. I
              think. So, after that we weren't spending every min-
              ute worrying about her or trying to get her out of trou-
              ble. So then, when all that was over it seemed like

there wasn't much else between us. I mean, we were a team when we were worried about Alicia and then it was like there was nothing else holding us together. If we didn't have Alicia to talk about it was like we didn't have anything.

Jane          You're saying the crisis with Alicia gave you a common purpose and when that was over there was nothing to take its place.

> *Jane summarizes what she just heard, as much for her own understanding as to clarify it for Sophie. Here she uses an EXISTENTIAL TACTIC that might help to strengthen the THERAPEUTIC ALLIANCE.*

Sophie        Exactly.

Jane          And how about before all that. When the kids were younger. Was it taking care of them that held you together? Was there more to the relationship than the parenting piece?

> *Jane begins to realize that her HYPOTHESIS is off the mark. It sounds now as though the marriage was more of a joint parenting operation than a love match.*

Sophie        I guess not. Dontrell was always out running around to all his stores, I was busy at home. Our sex life had become like an afterthought. Too busy. Too tired. We didn't have much in the way of a social life. Just things around the kids' school. You know, sports, school plays, PTA fundraisers. The kids always had their noses in front of a screen. The computer. Their phones. It seemed all right at the time, but I guess it wasn't.

Jane          Let's see if I've got the picture right. You're saying
              you and Dontrell had a relationship based on rais-
              ing the children, working together as a team, but not
              much in the way of feelings for each other. Is that
              right?

> *Jane again summarizes Sophie's ideas as
> a temporizing TACTIC. She has adopted a
> Rogerian type of EXISTENTIAL STRATEGY. Her
> purpose is to mark time while she clarifies
> what Sophie is saying.*

Sophie        Sounds sad when you put it that way but, yes, that's
              the way it was.

Jane          Okay. I get the picture now. So if it was a mar-
              riage based on mutual concern for the children, and
              the children are now on their own, or about to be
              when Jamal graduates, then there was no reason to
              stay together. And now you don't know what to do
              next.

> *Jane tries to come to terms with the failure
> of her HYPOTHESIS (suppressed anger toward
> Dontrell is the source of Sophie's collapse)
> by summing up the last 30 minutes while she
> tries to figure out how to proceed.*

Sophie        (Hesitantly) Yes.

Jane          Okay. Then let's talk about the question we were ask-
              ing before. What do you want to do now?

> *Jane backtracks to the prior discussion
> about Sophie's need for a new identity.*

Sophie      (Smirks) If I knew that I wouldn't need to be sitting here.

Jane        Well. I assume this isn't the first time you've thought about that. Can you share some of the ideas you've been considering?

> *Again, Jane feels like their discussion is just going through the motions, that Sophie is following the script but they're in the wrong play. She keeps going because she doesn't know what the alternative is.*

Sophie      (Throws up her hands) I thought I could go back to work. Find some kind of office job like I had before I got married. But that was boring when I was 18 and I don't think it would be any better now. So then I thought I should go to college, learn something useful. Do something I'd feel good about, you know?

Jane        College? What would you be interested in?

> *Sophie throws out a new topic so Jane goes with it.*

Sophie      Well, that's the thing. I don't know what I could do.

Jane        It sounds like you want to use college to prepare for getting an interesting job. What areas are you considering?

> *Jane, as usual, wants specifics, not general or vague ideas that don't advance the work.*

Sophie      Don't laugh. (Pauses) I'd like to be a social worker.

Jane        You think I would laugh?

*Jane wants to clarify whether Sophie expects
ridicule because of her own life experiences
or whether her expectation indicates
something negative about their THERAPEUTIC
ALLIANCE or an emerging TRANSFERENCE
issue. Her wording avoids a why question
(why would I laugh?).*

Sophie    Maybe I'm the one laughing. Me, a social worker?
          I'm a high school graduate. I'm black. It's 25 years
          since I've been in school. It all just seems too late.

Jane      You're worried the classes would be too hard for
          you?

          *Since it appears it was Sophie's own insecurity
          rather that an expectation of Jane's response,
          she continues to pursue the topic with a
          METACOMMUNICATION. Otherwise she would
          have needed to delve into why Sophie had an
          expectation that she, in particular, would laugh
          at her. Jane is not sure whether she should
          explore the agenda Sophie presents or focus on
          their therapeutic relationship, which remains
          an apparent weakness.*

Sophie    Not only that. I'd be this middle-aged African-
          American woman in a class full of teenagers. I'd
          stick out like a sore thumb.

                                          Time remaining
                                          5 minutes

Jane      Maybe not. People go back to school a lot these days.
          They take gap years then come back. They need new
          skills in this changing economy. There was a story in

the news recently about a grandmother who finally
went back to get her degree.

> *Jane makes a NORMATIVE statement. She
> treats Sophie's worry as a NEGATIVE
> OVERGENERALIZATION and tries to counter it
> with some opposing facts. A better approach
> might have been to elicit the details of the
> worry from Sophie, including what the effect
> of being an "African-American woman"
> might be as a factor in her plans.*

Sophie    Okay, but you need more than just college to be a social
worker. I looked it up. You need a Master's degree and
then some experience before you can get a license.

Jane    That's true.

> *Sophie has looked into this possible career
> path more carefully than Jane expected.
> She wonders if this is the unspoken agenda
> she has sensed in the background of their
> previous discussions.*

Sophie    You think I could do it?

Jane    What's important is what you think.

> *Jane does not want to be seen as Sophie's
> coach.*

Sophie    That's a cop out.

Jane    We can talk more about it next time, but our time is
up for today and we have to stop.

> *She acknowledges the importance of the
> discussion by suggesting it should be
> continued at the next visit.*

Sophie          (Stares at Jane thoughtfully, then gets up and walks out)

### Discussion

Jane's early work with Sophie has been both frustrating and unproductive. She found it unusual that Sophie countered her suggestion of six exploratory visits by asking for only three. That seemed like a red flag indicating that she was not very strongly committed to treatment, but Jane agreed to the shortened contract, thinking they could renegotiate if the initial meetings went well. Jane was unsure of the answer to the important question, what does the patient want from therapy? Her inductive conclusion, that Sophie could benefit from clarifying her self-identity in the face of all the family, social and biological changes she had encountered, even though she appeared to accept it, did not seem to engage her during the session. Now, Jane thinks all Sophie wants is someone to talk to or maybe she hopes Jane will be her (only) friend. What she wants to talk *about*, however, is still unidentified.

From the initial interview, Sophie's therapeutic alliance with Jane seemed to be somewhat weak. In this first therapy session, Jane was aware of making unusual efforts to engage Sophie more fully in the therapeutic process. These attempts included her efforts at social engagement and her persistence with topics such as the marriage and the career plans Sophie brought up. Jane wondered if Sophie felt less comfortable because Jane is not a member of the African-American minority. Whether matching race and gender improves psychotherapy outcomes remains an unsettled question (Ilagan & Heatherington, 2022). She realized she was trying harder than she otherwise might to engage Sophie in the exploration of what should have been topics of importance to her: not a hopeful sign.

Something seemed "off" about this session, but Jane was unable to discern what it was. Sophie discussed her relationship with her former husband, her daughter's behavioral problems in high school, her "empty nest" loneliness and her interest in training for a new career in social work. All of these topics were legitimate areas to examine, based on their treatment plan, but Sophie talked about them with less emotional investment than they would normally engender. It was almost as if she was playing the role of a therapy client without real interest in the process.

This phenomenon—a seeming detachment from the client's own life problems—might be expected from someone suffering from depression, where the person lacks the energy to invest the topics with the intensity they deserve, but Sophie is not clinically depressed. In the face of this apparent indifference, Jane went off on a tangent, pursuing her idea that the divorce left Sophie with unexpressed anger leading her into a paralysis. That hypothesis seems to have been incorrect. She then turned to another idea: having lost her identity as a wife and mother, Sophie now needs a new one.

Sophie showed the most interest in the discussion of a possible social work career. This idea fit in well with the chosen aim of treatment: consolidating a new self-identity. Jane declined, however, to adopt the role Sophie evidently expected, that of a life coach. That approach would involve setting up a plan of action with Jane helping her to achieve it. Sophie's disappointment about that placed them at odds as the session ends.

In short, this first therapy session left Jane with the uneasy feeling that she was missing something important without exactly knowing what it was.

## SESSION THREE

Sophie enters the office with a sheet of paper in her hand and takes her seat. She looks more put together in a collared blue shirt and pressed gray slacks. Jane notices that her hair is clean and darker and shows no gray; apparently she has been to a hairdresser during the last week. Jane wonders if perhaps this change in appearance mirrors an internal change for the better, suggesting at least a partial placebo effect.

Sophie    (Hesitantly) I want to ask you something. About what we talk about here. Is it completely confidential? I mean, nobody else could know. Isn't that right?

Jane      Yes, that true. I wouldn't tell anybody unless you asked me to or if a judge ordered me to.

> *Jane gives a brief but accurate answer. If Sophie wants more detail regarding patient–therapist confidentiality, Jane will provide it, but she waits to see what secret Sophie has decided to reveal.*

Sophie    (Thinks about this for a moment and nods her head) Okay. Well, I brought in something I'd like to read to you, if that's all right? I mean, this paragraph was like a revelation to me. It was my road to Damascus moment, if that doesn't sound too dramatic.[2] Shall I read it out loud?

Jane      It's up to you.

> *Jane tries to strengthen the* THERAPEUTIC ALLIANCE *by indicating that Sophie has power in the relationship. Not knowing what's coming, she tries to remain in a neutral stance.*

Sophie    Okay, well, here goes. (She looks down at the paper and then up at Jane) This is something I came across in a book. One of those mystery thriller type books. I read a lot of them, you know, it keeps my mind off my worries. (She turns her head and stares out the window, then turns back) Anyway, I was reading along and I came across this one paragraph. I read it over and over. I know it's crazy but it's like the author wrote it just for me. (Laughs and shakes her head) Like she just added this paragraph in the middle of the story for me to find it. So, here it is. (She brings the paper up and reads)

> *"There are certain pivotal moments in your life when you make a decision that will completely change the course of your existence. You might think you'll recognize those junctures when they arrive—that you'll perceive the importance of the moment, give your choice the proper gravitas and consideration, and then accept the consequences of your decision. And yet, so often, these choices happen unconsciously, unintentionally, a piling on of coincidence and circumstance rather than a moment of thoughtfulness. You aren't even aware they're happening."* (Brown J, 2022)

I saw this and I had to put the book down and go for a walk. I had to think it over and come to a decision. About my life and where I go from here.

Jane    May I see the page?

> *She wants to read it herself to be more clear on its significance.*

Sophie    (Hands it to Jane) Sure.

Jane    (After reading the passage carefully) Okay, I've got it. "Pivotal moments." What was yours?

> *Jane is eager to pursue this new development that promises to explain some of the confusion she had about the previous*

*session and wants to encourage Sophie to be as forthcoming as possible.*

Sophie      (Deep breath) What I'm going to tell you nobody else knows.

Jane        Okay. (She looks at Sophie with friendly expectation)
            *Jane is relieved at Sophie's decision to share a secret both because it indicates a stronger* THERAPEUTIC ALLIANCE *and because it might shed some light on whatever Sophie's hidden topic has been.*

Sophie      I'm... gay. I knew it when Dontrell asked me to marry him. But I said I would anyway. I mean, I'd never really been with another girl. I didn't know how. I didn't know anything. I was dating men and having sex with them—well, a few—thinking I'd get used to it. And then it was just like what I read to you. I made this gigantic decision—I said yes, I'd marry him—and I barely thought it through. It was... the thing was, then, to get married. (Begins to cry) That was success, you know. That's what girls were supposed to do. And Dontrell seemed like a nice guy and he was reliable. He had a job. This was even before he started franchising those McDonald's places. But I thought he'd be able to support us. So I agreed to get married and then the kids came along and I was busy with them. And I never realized what I was taking on. And now Dontrell's gone and the kids are going and here I am. (She dries her eyes and blows her nose)

Jane        (Nods) So, just to be clear. You've never been in a physical relationship with another woman?

*Jane wants to clarify whether Sophie is
sharing her hidden identity or whether
she has been leading a separate life with
sexual relationships other than her husband.
She also wants to convey that she is not
"shocked" by this news, since her question
implies acceptance with interest in the
details rather than any negative judgment.*

Sophie   Well, maybe once. I used to go to this summer camp
and then I stayed to be a junior counselor. And there
was one girl, Jenny, I was friends with and we'd you
know, kiss and roll around together. Never very serious. And then that was my last year at camp and I
never saw her again.

Time remaining
35 minutes

Jane   Your "pivotal moment" was when Dontrell proposed
and you said yes?

*Now she brings the discussion back to
Sophie's main point: that she made a
mistake in marrying Dontrell even though
the consequences of her choice only became
apparent as time went on.*

Sophie   It seemed like the right choice at the time. I was young.
I wasn't sure who I was. At least, getting married was a
thing to do, you know. When you're that age you don't
think very far ahead. But here I am 20 years later and
I've wasted all that time. Half my life. Over. And now
Dontrell's gone and the kids are grown. And now what?

Jane   I see what you mean. But I agree with you. When you
faced that pivotal moment and made that poor decision

you were only in your early twenties. When someone is that young they don't have the experience and the judgment to fully evaluate whatever choices they may face. In fact, we know that the human brain isn't fully developed until well after the teens, so that's another factor that weighs on young people when they have to make important decisions, even one as important as marriage. They don't have the full mental development they might need to make the best decision. Maybe that's one reason the divorce rate is so high.

> *Jane is uncertain about whether she should flag the* NEGATIVE OVERGENERALIZATION *(What about your children? Do you consider them a part of your wasting your life?) or whether she should continue to explore the new material Sophie has revealed, including why she has brought it up now. She settles for a (perhaps overly long)* NORMATIVE *and educational statement intended to ameliorate Sophie's self-blaming.*

Sophie    I wish I could go back and do it all over again. I don't know what I should do now.

Jane    Uh-huh.

> *A temporizing remark that ducks the implication that Jane should tell her what to do.*

Sophie    So now you know my secret. You're the only one I've ever told. (She looks expectantly at Jane) What should I do now?

Jane    Don't you think that's up to you?

*She uses a question instead of a statement ("That's up to you") to convey that she cannot solve Sophie's problem.*

Sophie   You don't have any ideas?

Jane     (Shakes her head)

         *She decides a non-verbal response is sufficient and conveys the stronger message.*

Sophie   So I'm on my own then. I'm in a bad place and you can't help me.

Jane     I can help you **decide** what you want to do with your life. I can't **tell** you what to do, if that's what you were asking.

         *Jane is careful to refer to the treatment contract and to renew her implied offer to help with what they agreed to work on together. She doesn't let Sophie's effort to guilt her into giving advice affect her therapeutic stance.*

Sophie   (Gets up and walks to the window. She stands looking out for several minutes) I don't want anyone else to know about me.

Jane     **Nobody** will hear about it from me.

         *Jane confirms her commitment to confidentiality.*

Sophie   (Turns and faces Jane) I was serious about what I said last time. I really would like to be a social worker.

                                                    Time remaining
                                                    25 minutes

Jane     What's your plan to get there?

*Jane accepts the change of topic by asking for details. Evidently, having shared her secret, Sophie now wants to leave it behind.*

Sophie    First I have to get a college degree. I thought about using one of those online programs. That way I don't have to sit in class with a bunch of children. But I don't know if that'll get me into a Master's program. I thought I'd go and talk to somebody at the university, somebody in the social work department, and find out if that'll work for me.

Jane    Sounds like you've already got your plan in place.

*Jane indirectly encourages her to say more about it. She avoids a direct question that would express doubt or signal to Sophie that Jane didn't believe she could do it.*

Sophie    (Returns to her seat and crosses a leg over her knee. Her pants cuff rides up, revealing what looks like a fresh tattoo.) It's a long-term commitment. Years. I'm already 46. (Shakes her head) By the time I qualify I'll be ready for retirement.

Jane    These days people work a lot longer than they used to. By the way, that looks like a new tattoo on your ankle.

*Jane makes another NORMATIVE statement that indirectly expresses her support for Sophie's plan. She asks about the tattoo to see what significance it has for Sophie in this new context.*

Sophie    It's a lotus. It stands for hope and new beginnings.

Jane    I see. So things must be coming together for you. About your future.

*Jane implies that the new tattoo is a good*
*sign in order to encourage her to say more*
*about her plans.*

Sophie    That's true. (Pauses) So you think I can do it? Social work?

Jane    I don't see any reason why not.

*Again, Jane tries to support the plan without*
*taking responsibility for it away from Sophie.*

Sophie    (Smiles) Yeah!

Jane    It sounds like you've been thinking about this for a while.

*Jane tries to encourage her to expand on*
*what makes this career choice appeal to her.*

Sophie    I have. For years. When Alicia was getting into all that trouble one of the people who helped us was a social worker. I was impressed. She just was so... self-contained. She knew what she was doing. She told us what we needed to do to help Alicia straighten out. She counseled Alicia herself for a while and that seemed to help her turn the corner. So I saw all that and I thought, I wish I could do that.

Jane    But yet you waited.

*She avoids a "why" question ("Why didn't*
*you do it?") that would imply disapproval.*

Sophie    I did.

Jane    How come?

*Again she avoids "why," but just barely.*

| Sophie | Like I told you, I didn't think I could. I looked into it, you know, college and then the postgraduate, and it just seemed like it was too long and I was too old. |
|---|---|

| Jane | What kind of grades did you get in school? |
|---|---|

*A FOUNDATIONAL question in preparation to explore the facts of the issue.*

| Sophie | Good ones. A's and B's. I was always a good student. I liked learning new stuff. I guess I was what you'd call a nerd. I would have **liked** to go to college but my family wasn't the college type. They said I should go to work. That I didn't need to spend four years piling up debt and not getting anything that would get me a better job. So that's what I did. I worked in that insurance office until I met Dontrell. That was another reason I married him. I wanted to get out of that office. (Shakes her head) God! How dumb was I? |
|---|---|

| Jane | It sounds like you'd be smart enough for the academics. |
|---|---|

*She makes a realistic observation intended to support Sophie's choice.*

| Sophie | Yeah? I hope you're right. |
|---|---|

Time remaining
15 minutes

| Jane | So then you've decided to pursue your degrees? |
|---|---|

*Jane wants to clarify the choice both for herself and for Sophie.*

| Sophie | I think so. |
|---|---|

Jane            All right. Well, you started off today telling me that you were gay. Should we talk more about that?

> *Again, Jane wants to show Sophie that she can use the therapy time as she thinks best. She does not direct her to talk about her sexual preference or indicate that she* **wants** *her to talk about it. She hopes that this collaborative stance will strengthen the* THERAPEUTIC ALLIANCE.

Sophie          I wanted somebody to know about it. I've never told anybody before. Nobody ever talked about it. Now, you know, it's all over the news. Gay Pride Day and marches and same sex marriage. It seems more acceptable. (Frowns) But I don't know if it really is. The people with the loudest voices are getting heard, but the rest of the country hasn't changed. So I thought I'd tell you and see what happened.

Jane            It felt safer to tell me.

> *Jane makes an empathetic statement to see if Sophie will say more about her fears.*

Sophie          It did. And I thought you were okay with it.

Jane            I am. But you're right. Not everybody would be. What do you think would be your family's reaction?

> *Jane suspects that the family is the source of Sophie's conflict about her sexuality and introduces it as the most significant issue for Sophie.*

Sophie          Not good. My brothers wouldn't like it. Well, I know John wouldn't. He's the one who drives for UPS. My brother, Sonny, he's in the Army. He might have gotten some new ideas.

Jane     And your parents?

*She expects the parents are the most important barriers to Sophie's "coming out."*

Sophie   Wouldn't like it all. They'd probably pretend it never happened. Either that or they'd stop talking to me. I mean, the divorce was bad enough but that… it would be the end.

Jane     The end.

*She echoes Sophie to encourage her to say more.*

Sophie   Yeah. I could never… (She puts her head in her hands and rocks gently back and forth)

Jane     Well, suppose you met a woman, you liked her, it developed into a strong mutual relationship and you decided to get married again.

*Jane uses this hypothetical as a FOUNDATION to confront the risk Sophie feels from her parents finding out about her.*

Sophie   (Looking up) Whoa, that would be a blockbuster! I doubt my family would even come to the wedding. I don't think I'd even tell them.

Jane     Here's a thought: does the way you see your family's attitude, could that be why you grew up thinking badly of yourself about being gay?

*Now she uses Sophie's recognition as a basis for offering an interpretive question.*

Sophie     Yeah. All that talk about fags and dykes. I see
           what you mean. (Grimaces) But still, that's not a
           surprise, is it? I mean, what parents want to hear
           their child isn't normal? Isn't going to ever give
           them grandchildren or be able to boast about their
           accomplishments?

Jane       I don't know about all parents but what's important
           is how you think about your parents. How do you
           know they would both reject you? And is it the same
           for your mother as it would be with your father? Are
           they always in lock step?

           *Jane rejects the OVERGENERALIZATION and
           tries to focus Sophie on her own parents.*

Sophie     I could never tell them. I just couldn't. What would I
           say, "Hey, Ma, I'm a lezzy"?

Jane       I'm not suggesting you tell them, although I'm not
           saying don't tell them either. What I think it would
           be helpful to consider is what I said before. How
           you feel about yourself: to what extent did growing
           up in your particular family shape the way you feel
           about yourself? Isn't that what's important? Isn't
           that what you need to move forward? If you stop
           thinking about yourself using your parents' ideas
           you might be able to accept the way you feel without
           being ashamed.

           *Jane tries to sum up what she wants Sophie
           to get out of this discussion. Since she chose
           to share her secret with her, Jane thinks
           she has an unusual opportunity to modify
           Sophie's self-image and free her up from the
           self-imposed shame she has been carrying
           throughout her adult life.*

| Sophie | That's easy for you to say. They're still my parents. I can't get away from that. |
|---|---|

| Jane | Do you see them much? Do they live nearby? Do they visit? |
|---|---|

> *Jane wants to lay a FOUNDATION to discuss her current relationship with her parents.*

| Sophie | Not much. They live, like, four hours away. We used to see them more when the kids were little but since the divorce and the kids are older we don't. I mean, I don't. |
|---|---|

Time remaining
5 minutes

| Jane | So, maybe we're not talking about your parents the way they are now—older, retired, out of your life— maybe we're talking about them when you were growing up, when they had a much stronger influence on you. |
|---|---|

> *Jane wants to introduce the concept of Sophie's parents as INTROJECTED OBJECTS that might be modified by later experience.*

| Sophie | (Shakes her head) I don't think they're any different now. |
|---|---|

| Jane | Well, I don't know them, of course, but I'd be surprised if they hadn't learned **anything** in the last 25 years. Most people do. But that's not the point. What I meant was that children take in what they see as their parents' values, ideas… and their prejudices when they're young. And those things can stay with the child long after they've grown up. |
|---|---|

> *Jane starts with a NORMATIVE assertion but follows it with an educational statement about INTROJECTION that she hopes will help Sophie think about how she views her parents and their biases.*

Sophie     (Slowly, as if she's considering it) Okay.

Jane       Maybe we can talk more about that next time.
> *Jane is preparing to end the session.*

Sophie     Yeah. About that. I think I'm going to stop at this point. Maybe think about things for a while on my own.

Jane       I thought we agreed on three trial sessions!
> *Jane is caught off guard by this sudden development and weakly reminds Sophie of the treatment contract. A better response would have been to ask for Sophie's reasons behind the decision but Jane is too startled to think of that.*

Sophie     (Firmly) Well, I think I'm good now. I'll let you know if I want to come again.

Jane       Okay. It's certainly up to you. I hope your plans work out.
> *Jane tries to recover and wish her the best.*

Sophie     Thanks. (She gets up and leaves the office)

Jane       (To herself) Well, that was a surprise!

## Discussion

The marked contrast between this session and the previous meeting raises several questions that Jane has insufficient data to fully answer.

- How real are the changes that occurred over only a week between visits?
- Was the sudden improvement a so-called "flight into health," a rapid apparent improvement based on no real internal change that may or may not continue? (Train, 1953).
- What allowed Sophie to form a well-developed plan for her to proceed with her life?
- How well will she be able to deal with problems arising from her sexual identity?
- Will she be able to persevere along the long, difficult road to her new career as a social worker?

Absent a third meeting and the possibility of additional therapy, these questions will remain unexplored.

That Sophie found a passage in a novel that resonated so strongly with her was an act of serendipity, a lucky chance, that catalyzed the breakthrough in her brief therapy. She plunged right into a discussion of her unexpressed sexuality and tied it into her regretted decision to marry a man. With the secret out she was able to talk about herself more freely and seemed to respond to Jane's therapeutic ideas, such as the early influence of parental attitudes. She was able to reach Jane's projected outcome of consolidating a new identity. She acquired a new tattoo that celebrates her growth and looks to the future.

Sophie did most of the work in this second session. She got what she wanted from therapy: someone to talk to, a sounding board that she could use to test out not only her "secret" but also her ambitious educational goals. Most of the improvement was due to Sophie's use of the therapy time to give voice to her problems, such as her shame, her loneliness and her fears of the future. Jane's efforts to help her clarify her feelings and to make new plans played a relatively minor role. Sophie was able to use her as a non-judgmental listener to clarify ideas that, unexpressed, were unexamined and non-operational. Not the most satisfying exercise from Jane's point of view, but she'll take it as a win.

## Notes

1 In *Games People Play*, Eric Berne describes the transactional "game," *Why Don't You Yes But* (WDYYB) as one person asking another for advice only to find fault with every suggestion (Berne, 1969).
2 A reference to a biblical story: Saul, a critic of Jesus who is traveling to Damascus, is converted to the disciple, Paul, by a blinding flash of light and hearing the voice of Jesus.

## References

Berne, E. (1969). *Games People Play*. Knopf Doubleday.

Brown, J. (2022). I'll Be You. *Random House*, 276.

Ilagan, G. S., & Heatherington, L. (2022). Advancing the understanding of factors that influence client preferences for race and gender. *Counseling Psychology Quarterly*, 35(3), 694–717.

Train, G. F. (1953). Flight into health. *American Journal of Psychotherapy*, 7(3), 463.

# Martin

## An Isolated Young Researcher

### Referral

Martin is a patient in Jane's private practice. He was referred by his primary practitioner with the comment, "needs more therapy." Chief complaint: "I am all screwed up." What he wants from therapy, he says, is "a normal life."

### History

Martin is 26 years old, single and recently employed as a research scientist at a large pharmaceutical company. While a postgraduate student in another city, he applied to a psychoanalytic clinic and was treated by a psychoanalyst-in-training four times a week. Now, however, he has come for once-weekly psychotherapy because he can't afford any more psychoanalysis, his new job won't allow him more time, and also because he felt he had not gained much help from his previous treatment. He has mild-to-moderate social anxiety that is unchanged by his prior treatment. He has acquaintances but not friends and no significant history of dating or relationships with women. Jane also noted his intellectualism and rigidity. So far, his new job has been going well.

Martin is an only child raised in an intact family. His father is a pharmacist, and was an emotionally distant, rigid and perfectionistic parent. Martin thinks he resembles his father in many ways. His mother is an early education teacher, working with both first and second grade. She was the warmer, more supportive parent, although because of her work she was not as available as he would

DOI: 10.4324/9781003353003-9

have liked. Martin was always one of the top students in school, a status he feels was a barrier to friendships in grade school and high school ("I was always known as 'the brain'").

In college, he remained socially withdrawn and only distantly friendly with roommates.

In social situations, he usually feels self-conscious and awkward, expecting to be judged unfavorably by others. He is aware of thinking how what he might say would be received before he allows himself to speak, so that in conversation he seems to pause unnecessarily and lacks spontaneity. His hobbies, both in high school and college, were chess and video gaming. He tried marijuana but disliked the loss of control he felt. He used alcohol to help in social situations but avoided heavy drinking. He majored in biochemistry and went on to get a PhD in molecular biology.

In graduate school, he was friendly with a female student—they worked in the same lab—but they did not date. Martin thought the woman was interested in him, but he did not feel drawn to her or find her physically attractive. He has not had a sexual relationship but masturbates and watches online pornography.

## Mental Status Examination

Martin presents as well-groomed and appropriately but casually dressed: an open-collar shirt and cotton trousers with New Balance running shoes. He is smart and articulate, but his demeanor is detached. He is emotionally reserved with little affect and he sometimes appears grim. His judgment is overly critical and rigid. His speech is mildly pressured and his mood seems somewhat anxious. At times, he has vague thoughts of death, and believes "no one would care," but he denies suicidal ideation. Sleep and appetite are normal.

## Formulation

Martin seems unable to progress from adolescence to young adulthood, a developmental step Erikson characterized as a struggle between isolation and intimacy (Erikson, 1959). Graduate school served to protect him because it delayed his having to confront this developmental transition. His social isolation seems both a contributing cause of his loneliness and also is his mechanism for avoiding anxiety and the risk to his self-esteem presented by social encounters and relationships with women.[1] His rigidity, intellectualism and need for control have no doubt been helpful to him as a research scientist, but these traits contribute to his isolation as well. His motivation for therapy is high. His motivation for change is moderate.

(Formulation Category: Developmental, possibly Transactional)

**Treatment Plan**

The *aim* is to help him resume progress in the developmental step of moving from isolation toward greater intimacy, both in the sphere of general friendships and the possible choice of a life partner that might result from having affection-based relationships with women. To achieve this outcome, three *goals* are needed: modify some of his personality traits; increase his social interactions overall (which means reducing his social anxiety); and initiate one or more meaningful relationships with women. While cognitive therapy may be helpful to deal with the social anxiety, and may also be useful for developing more meaningful relationships, a psychodynamic *strategy* seems the better modality for the other goals. This choice is based not only on the need to modify his personality traits but also because, after years of psychoanalysis, it may be the type of therapy with which he is most familiar and comfortable.

The initial meeting began with an assessment and then discussion of what therapy might reasonably achieve. Jane believes she has a treatment contract with Martin that includes a focus on his social anxiety and his interpersonal relationships. Unstated, but important in Jane's plan, is a goal of modifying those traits that contribute to his other difficulties. Session Two initiates the treatment proper.

**SESSION TWO**

Martin arrives at 4:06 PM for his 4:00 PM session. He wears a grey sweater over an open-neck white dress shirt and jeans with ankle boots. Jane assumes this is what he wears to the lab, since he has come directly from work to the session.

Martin          (Taking his seat) Sorry I'm late.

                                              Time remaining
                                              39 minutes

Jane            (Nods but doesn't speak)

> *Martin's tone is perfunctory, a conversational gambit rather than actual regret. Jane chooses not to make an issue of it since (1) it's only six minutes, (2) Martin's pro forma apology shows he isn't focused on it and (3) the lateness is not yet part of a pattern. Perhaps this SYMPTOMATIC ACT signifies his need for control (at least of the time) or it might presage a beginning resistance. It does not yet require an intervention.*

Martin          (He stares up at a corner of the ceiling) So, I've been thinking about women.

Jane            Women?

> *Jane notes his use of the general category, "women," an abstraction, rather than any particular person. She uses a single interlocutory word in place of a longer question to indicate she'd like to hear more about the topic without being specific about what she wants to hear, as that might distort his response. Often, the slightest indication of interest by the therapist, even simply clearing the throat, serves to focus the patient on topic.*

Martin          Yep. I think I've figured out why I don't like them.

Jane        You don't like any of them?

> *Jane wonders if this non-verbal behavior*
> *(avoiding looking at someone he's speaking to)*
> *reflects his previous psychoanalytic therapy,*
> *where he lay on a couch and didn't make eye*
> *contact with the therapist. Again, Jane tries to*
> *flag the abstraction, the generalization. Does*
> *he include her or, based on his experience with*
> *the invisible psychoanalyst, is she merely a*
> *blank listener?*

Martin      No. Look at the way they dress. (Now he stares
            out the window, still not talking to her directly)
            Everything's uncovered. Their chests, their arms,
            their legs. They go around half-naked and then
            they expect you to take them seriously? (Clears his
            throat) They do everything possible to attract atten-
            tion to their boobs, but then they resent it when you
            stare at them. If they don't want you to look why do
            they wear a push-up bra and low necklines? And the
            makeup. They make their faces like circus clowns.
            They dye their hair. They don't want you to see what
            they really look like. And, you know, now they think
            hair dyes can cause breast cancer. Serves them right,
            the phonies.

Jane        Are you really as angry about this as you sound?

> *With this METACOMMUNICATIVE question Jane*
> *tries to help Martin recognize the emotional*
> *component to his intellectual arguments. He*
> *implies that he doesn't want a relationship with*
> *a woman, but it sounds like "sour grapes."*

Martin      (Glances at Jane and then away) No, I'm not angry.
            Just making observations.

Jane            "Serves them right" sounds like more than an observation.

> *Martin has started his first treatment session with her, a woman, by announcing he dislikes women! Jane wonders about this unusual gambit. Is he telling her he resents her as a woman? Is he intellectualizing about the topic to defend against his anxiety around women (including her)? Is it another attempt at control by setting the session's agenda? Is arriving with a plan of what to talk about a reflection of his previous treatment with the silent, out of sight psychoanalyst? Does he diminish his social anxiety by having a prepared speech to begin his interaction with her? Jane has no answers as yet to any of these questions, but these ideas are HYPOTHESES she can explore as therapy progresses.*

Martin          (Still not making eye contact) It's just a logical conclusion. I mean, what are you supposed to think when they stick pieces of metal all over their faces and ugly tattoos everywhere else? They look like they belong to some aboriginal tribe that's been discovered living in the rainforest. It's like they've regressed into some primitive level of human behavior.

> Time remaining
> 35 minutes

Jane            Are you thinking of anyone in particular?

> *Jane wants to confront Martin's intellectual style and the abstract approach he uses to distance himself from his feelings. Who is the actual object of this diatribe?*

| Martin | No. (He glances at her again and then resumes watching the window) I was watching a news show on TV. The men are dressed in suits. They wear ties. The women are in bare-shouldered dresses. They look like they're going to a bar to get laid. It's disgusting. |

| Jane | (With emphasis) Disgusting! |

*When he finally reveals an emotion, it seems over the top. Jane highlights it for him.*

| Martin | Absolutely. Sex for women is an asset. They offer sex for some kind of payment. Maybe it's buying them dinner. Maybe it's a piece of jewelry. Maybe it's a marriage proposal. And then the marriage breaks up and they get half of everything the guy has, and they did nothing to earn it. Except provide sex. Alimony is just deferred payment for sex. They always have to get something in return. (Pauses) Or maybe not always. Sometimes they'll offer it as a gift. Then they say to the guy he's going to get lucky. Why is that? Why is it always the man who's lucky, never the woman? It's because they're giving the guy sex supposedly without requiring payment in advance! Of course, if you look at it more closely, there's usually some kind of quid pro quo. Maybe in the future. Something to be claimed later. "I gave you sex so now you owe me." It's always a trade. They barter it. They have to get something for it, now or later. They're all secret prostitutes. |

| Jane | It sounds like you've been giving this a lot of thought. |

*Martin fails to pick up on the "disgust" and immediately returns to his abstract argument. Jane again makes a METACOMMUNICATION that suggests this topic is more important*

*than just an editorial essay. She avoids a
"why" question (for example, "Why are you
telling me this?") as she tries to find out the
reason Martin has launched into this topic
and with so much heat.*

Martin       Not really.

Jane         Doesn't the fact that you brought it up first thing
             today mean that it's something you feel is important
             to you?

             *Jane believes this topic has a more personal
             significance for him, so rather than letting
             it go, she challenges his denial and invites
             further discussion.*

Martin       (Looking at the floor) No. I was just telling you what
             was on my mind.

Jane         That's what you would do with Dr. Parker, right? Say
             whatever came into your mind?

             *Dr. Parker was the trainee-psychoanalyst
             Martin saw before he moved to his new job.
             His avoidance of eye contact has persisted and
             is becoming an obstruction to their therapeutic
             communication, so it needs to be addressed.
             She makes an educated guess that it derives
             from his prior psychoanalysis: lying on a
             couch producing "free associations" with the
             analyst out of sight behind him.*

Martin       Sure.

Jane         I notice that you're not looking at me while you're
             talking. Is that something from Dr. Parker, too?

*By describing his non-verbal behavior,
Jane hopes this* METACOMMUNICATION *will
make him aware of its strangeness and then
perhaps to change it.*

Martin      I thought that was supposed to help. You know, get in touch with my unconscious or something.

Jane      I think we should focus more on what your current problems are.

*Jane believes a good rule for psychotherapy
is "stay on the surface" and let underlying
issues develop naturally. This comment is
meant to convey that idea to Martin.*

Martin      (Now he looks at her) That's not what I'm used to. It was different with Dr. Parker.

Jane      Well, that was a different kind of therapy. We can make more progress if we focus on the things we agreed to work on.

*Part of the treatment contract is the
methodology that will be used to pursue the
treatment* GOALS. *Jane did not make that
explicit in her earlier discussions.*

Martin      (Stares) Like what?

Jane      One of those things was to help you with personal relationships, and how you feel about women might be part of that.

*An educational statement. Jane reminds him
of the* THERAPEUTIC CONTRACT *and the way it
differs from his previous therapy.*

Martin       (Bitterly) Hah! There **are** no women in my life.

Jane         Could that be because you're so angry at half the
             world's population? Could it be your suspicion that
             every single one of them is a dishonest schemer out
             to trap you?

             *Jane avoids including herself: she does not
             say, for example: "...because you're so
             angry at us." Martin's bitter tone suggests
             an emotional basis for this diatribe. Jane
             hopes her response, engaging him directly,
             will reinforce his willingness to show his
             feelings. She puts her explanation in the form
             of questions to invite his attention without
             making it a challenge. She does three things
             with this intervention. She RENAMES Martin's
             "intellectual" position using emotional
             words like "angry" and "suspicion." She
             makes a connection between Martin's
             intellectual approach and his more personal
             problem of social isolation. She confronts
             him with the negative OVERGENERALIZATION
             behind his apparent distress.*

Martin       (Shrugs) Hey, I'm just telling it like it is. It's biology.
             It's evolution. Women are programmed to get a mate
             and make sure he stays around to support her and her
             offspring. Sex is their means to accomplish that.

Jane         So there are no women in your life because of Darwin?

             *Martin immediately resumes his intellectual
             defense. Jane uses a RHETORICAL device
             to reflect his idea back to him in an
             exaggerated way that undermines his
             abstract argument.*

Martin      (Chuckles) Hey, that's good. I hadn't thought of it that way.

Time remaining<br>25 minutes

Jane        So what's this all about?

> *Martin's laughter seems to recognize the sophistry of his argument. Jane takes advantage of the shift away from speechifying to ask again what provoked it.*

Martin      (Looking directly at her) Well, it's something at work. Turns out I got a warning from HR about (he uses his fingers to make air quotes) "sexual harassment."

Jane        Oh?

> *Jane uses this tell-me-more response to indicate her non-judgmental interest. Again, one word suffices.*

Martin      Yeah, I was surprised. Turns out I was harassing somebody and I didn't even know it.

Jane        Who was it that complained about you?

> *"Somebody" is still an abstract way of avoiding the feelings in the situation. Jane asks for a concrete response, an actual person.*

Martin      One of the lab assistants. She has this green hair. Like lime Jell-O green. Actually, I think it looks nice, but I've been teasing her about it. You know, like: Hey, did you water that thing today?

Jane        What's her name, this lab assistant?

*Martin still hasn't named the person who
complained, as if it wasn't personal. Jane
persists in asking for particulars. She could
have used a* METACOMMUNICATION *to point
out how he avoided them but her need for
more facts outweighs the benefit of a more
general observation.*

Martin    Bettina. That's her name.

Jane    Okay, and you wanted to get Bettina's attention?

> *She repeats the woman's name to solidify the
> discussion about the specific person.*

Martin    (He looks away again) Yeah, maybe…

Jane    And how did Bettina react, when you were teasing
her?

> *She puts the focus on emotion. Can he
> recognize what others are feeling? She uses
> Martin's term, teasing, to maintain focus on
> the event and to match his* DICTION.

Martin    Oh, she would just give a little smile. She didn't
really look at me.

Jane    Do you think she was uncomfortable with being ver-
bally assaulted?

> *Martin still doesn't appreciate the impact
> of his teasing on the woman's feelings. She
> tries a more direct approach,* NAMING *it with
> a stronger word. (She could also have said:
> threatened, insulted, harassed, angered, etc.)
> to help him recognize his effect on Bettina.*

Martin      (Grimaces) Obviously, if she made a complaint. And now they transferred her to a different lab.

Jane      That sounds pretty serious.

> *Jane characterizes the situation, since he seems to shrug it off. Martin seems unaware of his own stimulus power: that the response he might get from another person is caused by how he acts toward them.*

Martin      Well, I'm on probation. If it happens again, they told me, I could be fired.

Jane      Fired!

> *She picks up the word "fired" to acknowledge how serious it is.*

Martin      (Rolls his eyes) Yeah. Well, one thing, I'm not talking to any of the women employees. That's for sure.

Jane      Because you don't know how they'd take it? But don't you have to interact with the women at work **about** the work that you're doing?

> *Martin responds with a childish and probably unrealistic response. He focuses on his own risk without recognizing his effect on his female coworkers. Jane challenges the solution as unrealistic.*

Martin      (Shrugs) It could happen, but now that they transferred Bettina out of my lab, everybody else is a man.

Jane      Okay, maybe that solves the immediate problem, but what about the bigger issue: how to develop personal relationships. With women **and** men, actually. That was something you wanted to accomplish from this therapy.

> *She reminds him of a treatment* GOAL. *So far, the theme of the session seems to be Martin's pattern of viewing women as abstractions, a homogeneous group of strange and dangerous beings.*

Martin      (Frowns) Yeah? And how am I supposed to do that?

Jane      Well, first you have to want to.

> *Jane chooses to respond to his question with a challenge: is he motivated to change? She implies that she can't tell him what to do; he has to find the solution on his own.*

Martin      (Sits up straight) I do want to. I wanted to ask Bettina out on a date, before she complained about me.

Jane      What made you hesitate?

> *She presumes his hesitation reflected his social anxiety, but she asks the question to help focus on his feelings.*

Martin      (Embarrassed grin) Well, fear. I was afraid she'd say no.

Jane      So, teasing her about her hair was a way of testing the water?

> *Martin acknowledges a feeling, fear, a breakthrough for him. Jane's suggestion* INTERPRETS *his motivation as a question that asks him to expand on how he felt.*

Martin    I guess so. Yeah. But I wasn't getting a clear signal back.

Jane      You didn't pick up on the signal, did you? What she seems to have been signaling was that she didn't like you teasing her. Or, maybe, that she wanted to be treated as a fellow professional, rather than as an object of ridicule.

> *"Picking up signals" is a form of empathy. Martin apparently either lacks it, which would suggest a SOCIOPATHIC trait, or he doesn't exercise that mental function, a more hopeful possibility. Jane tries to provide examples for him to see which of the two it might be.*

Martin    You think I was ridiculing her?

Jane      The question is, what did Bettina think?

> *She avoids giving her opinion and again focuses on Martin's empathy or lack of it. Another response would have been to ask, "Can you think of any other reasons for Bettina's reaction?" Jane is unsure at this point, however, if he is capable of coming up with alternative reasons.*

Martin    (Shrugs) I guess I didn't think about that... I did see she wasn't too thrilled with me. She'd frown or turn away. I ignored that.

Jane      Maybe what you thought of as friendly teasing, Bettina took to be hostility. She must have felt threatened to go so far as to take it to the HR people and get herself transferred.

*He does seem to have the capacity to empathize. Jane chooses to spell it out for him. The risk is that Martin could come to rely on her to "translate" social situations for him instead of learning to do it himself.*

Martin     Oh, I see. When you put it like that, yeah, maybe I did screw things up.

Jane       So, how do you think it went wrong?

*She keeps the focus on his behavior, asking for him to be introspective.*

Martin     (Shakes his head) God, I don't know.

Jane       Could it be that you didn't think about Bettina as another person, but just someone out to trap you with sex, one of those predatory women you're so worried about?

*Feeling a little frustrated that he doesn't focus on his internal attitude, she tries to make it overt for him. While it may help to make this connection, it means he doesn't have to do the work himself, which would be the more useful result.*

Martin     That's what you think?

Time remaining
15 minutes

Jane       You're the one who said that before, that all women are using sex to get what they want.

*Defensively, he "forgets" his earlier rant. She reminds him.*

| | |
|---|---|
| Martin | (Frowns) Yeah, but I wasn't thinking that about Bettina. I liked her. |
| Jane | Apparently, you didn't get that across to her. |
| | *She still feels frustrated at his lack of insight and makes it obvious. She could have made her point more usefully with a question; such as, "What do you think Bettina was feeling?" Jane wonders if she has been maneuvered into defending women in reaction to Martin's earlier criticisms.* |
| Martin | Yeah, no shit. |
| Jane | Is that a problem you've had with other women? |
| | *Now she tries to use it more productively by asking him to generalize and to consider the pattern of his behavior.* |
| Martin | (Raised eyebrows) Other women? No one's reported me to HR before. |
| Jane | I'm asking about women you might have dated in the past or even other women you've been in class with or worked with. |
| | *That she has to spell it out for him suggests that he is being deliberately dense as a way to avoid her question.* |
| Martin | Yeah, no. I haven't had this problem before. |
| Jane | I don't know about that. Somehow I doubt Bettina was the first woman who misunderstood your interest. What about the ones you dated in college? What happened with them? |

*Her first two statements reveal her frustration with his answer and would have been better avoided. Again a question like, "Really? Bettina was the first?" might be more productive.*

Martin       (Irritated) It never worked out. Either they didn't like me or I didn't like them.

Jane         What was it about them you didn't like?

*He gives an explanation that doesn't actually address the question. Jane focuses on his feelings toward the women rather than the unknown issue of what they felt.*

Martin       (Chuckles) Mostly that they didn't seem to like **me**.

Jane         Can you pick one of them as an example?

*He avoids his feelings and makes a joke about theirs, a way of deflecting from the topic. He has been trying to avoid this topic throughout the session, beginning perhaps with arriving late. His tirade about "women" now seems like another avoidance ploy. Still, it feels to Jane like he's willing to deal with this issue, so she persists. She tries to make it as specific as possible.*

Martin       I don't... I hardly remember them. Well, one of them. Her name was Madison... Maddy. We went out for a few weeks, off and on, and then she ghosted me.

Jane         Any idea what made her do that?

*She picks up on the rejection rather than asking for more detail about their*

> *relationship, the details of which might have laid a better FOUNDATION for the discussion.*

Martin        (Shakes his head) No.

Jane          Must've been something. What happened the last time you saw her?

> *She needs more detail in order to explore how Martin contributed to this unsatisfactory outcome. He seems reluctant to discuss this relationship. A METACOMMUNICATION would be helpful here. For example, "Do you want to talk about this topic? It seems like you're having a hard time with it."*

Martin        Hmm. So long ago. (Looks up at the ceiling) We went to a party, I think. Yeah, a party in the dorm. I had a few drinks. I was a little buzzed so I could talk to people. Then, after that we were walking around outside and we got into a kind of argument, about where things stood with us. We'd had maybe three dates by then. So, she wanted to know about that because I was talking to another girl at the party and maybe I was annoying her. I'm not really sure.

Jane          When you said you annoyed her, what do you think Maddy was feeling at that moment?

> *Martin doesn't seem to recognize that Maddy could have been jealous of his attentions to another woman.*

Martin        It was a girl I knew from one of my classes. I don't even know what we talked about. Homework, maybe. Something stupid. (Shakes his head) It was like she wanted a ring on her finger or we'd break up. And I sure wasn't thinking that far ahead.

| Jane | Maddy said that? That she wanted to get engaged? |

*Jane doubts that Maddy wanted a marriage proposal on their fourth date. She wants him to distinguish between what actually happened and his improbable excuse.*

| Martin | Not exactly. (Sits forward in his chair) I mean, she didn't ask for a ring or anything. Look, I was a kid in college. I was horny. What I was probably thinking was whether she'd have sex with me. That's what kids think about. Not getting married to the girl. |

| Jane | Were you having sex? |

*She poses a question even though she expects the answer to be no. His generalization, "what kids think," is irrelevant, so she keeps the focus on him.*

| Martin | No, we weren't. And before you ask, no I haven't. I'm still a virgin. |

| Jane | Why do you think that is? |

*He has made an important admission, something about which he feels frustration and shame, so Jane shifts the discussion to it. Her "why" question is simply a request for information.*

| Martin | Beats me. Are girls even interested in sex? Apparently not with me. (He stops speaking and looks down at the floor) I just never get that far with the girls I go out with, and there aren't very many of them. I wanted to have sex with Maddy but she didn't. |

Jane    You said you kind of ignored her at the party. Do you think she felt hurt by that? Maybe abandoned?

>    *Since he is reluctant to pursue the new topic, and even stops talking and then returns to the college incident, Jane leaves the discussion of his "virginity" for a possible future exploration.*

Martin    Really?

Jane    Could this have been another case where you didn't think about how the other person might feel? Like Bettina in the lab?

>    *She offers the INTERPRETATION that how women (and others) respond to him might reflect his own insensitive behavior, but uses the two specific instances to make it more relevant to him.*

Martin    (Throws up his hands) Why are these girls so sensitive? Christ! It's like you have to tiptoe around all the time.

Jane    Is it the women or is it you not picking up how the other person feels?

>    *His emotional response indicates the INTERPRETATION was on target. She restates it as a step in the process of WORKING THROUGH.*

Martin    I'm not getting the signals again?

Time remaining
5 minutes

Jane    Seems like you're not.

*His response shows that he is beginning to accept the idea that his limited social skills and his self-absorption are contributing to his failed relationships.*

Martin    I guess I'll have to work on that.

Jane    How will you do that?

*By not accepting the generalization, she hopes he will continue to consider new behavior.*

Martin    (Hangs his head) Shit, I don't know!

Jane    Most people have a kind of mental filter. They review what they want to say before they say it out loud. They try to imagine how their words might come across to the other person. Is that something you do?

*She knows from his history that he does this as a manifestation of his social anxiety. In fact, he is overly aware of other people's possible perceptions of him, expecting them to form a negative opinion. She wants him to use his already existing habit of self-scrutiny as a pathway to behavior change.*

Martin    Yeah. Well, usually. Sometimes I just say what I think. Besides, how can you know what the other person is thinking?

Jane    It sounds like you knew what Bettina was feeling but you ignored it and teased her anyway. Maybe we should think about it this way. Teasing is a two-edged sword. There's the humorous side of it and then there's the hostile side. You say something hurtful to the other person hoping they'll take it as a joke. Isn't that right?

> *She spells it out for him. Now that he recognizes the problem she can offer him a tool to deal with it. Also, she again uses his word, teasing, to maintain appropriate DICTION.*

Martin    I guess so. I wasn't thinking about it that way. But, yeah, I guess I was a little hostile. She was ignoring me and that made me angry.

Jane    Based on how she reacted, going to HR, she understood the hostility part better than you did. Maybe you were so focused on your own feelings, including your interest in dating her, that you didn't pay enough attention to how she might feel about what you were doing. You ignored the cues she was giving you until she felt she had to take drastic action.

> *Martin seems to have gained a significant insight, but further work will be needed to translate the insight into a meaningful change in his behavior toward women. The session is about to end, so Jane summarizes a bit to try to solidify the gains they made.*

Martin    Yeah, you're right.

Jane    Our time is up for today and we have to stop.

Martin    Okay.

### *Discussion*

Jane found herself unusually active in this session, even telling Martin things about "women" he might better have come to realize on his own. In part, her active role was a response to the passive, silent psychoanalyst that Martin's four years in analysis led him to expect.[2] In part, Martin baited her (probably without conscious thought) to take an adversarial position to his views about women. That may turn out to be how he operates, provoking people as a way of making contact with them. Although she failed to recognize it at the time, she will be on the alert for it in the future.

This session made some progress toward the treatment goals. Jane's steady focus on helping Martin identify his feelings and modify his intellectualizing was significant. She did not, for example, ask him for an account of the meeting with the HR representative or the conditions of his probation, topics that would divert the focus from his emotional responses.

She achieved a minor breakthrough through the use of a rhetorical device when she asked if his problem was Darwinian, exaggerating for effect, and Martin responded with self-aware laughter and only then revealed he had been put on probation for possible sexual harassment. This moment was a turning point in the session, which then could focus on his interaction with a female coworker instead of his hostile ramblings about women in general.

Jane avoided an alternative approach in which she could have labeled his attitude as "misogynistic." Naming his anti-woman speech with a negative label might have allowed him to back off and review his opinions more objectively, but it would not have focused as directly on the treatment goals. (If she had used that term, the diction involved, the choice of "misogyny," would be consistent with Martin's intelligence and level of education.)

## SESSION THREE

Martin arrives early and paces the waiting room. He is apparently well trained by his four years on the couch with Dr. Parker. Another patient, arriving early, might knock on the door or even walk in. Both actions would be a boundary violation. Jane opens the office door to allow him in and Martin enters the office with a bounce in his step. He seems to be in an unusually good mood. He sits forward in his chair and makes direct eye contact with Jane.

Time remaining
45 minutes

Martin    (Smugly) Lemme tell you what happened at work today. We had these visitors from the London office? Three Brits. And we're sitting around at lunch and one of them says, he says, you Americans don't know how to speak English (using his fingers to indicate air quotes) "properly." And then he gives us an example that we say **dumb** when we should say **stupid**, because "dumb" means "mute," right? He says this with, like, a sneer, the arrogant little prick. So I said, well, he was a guest in our country and it would be only polite to help him out with his language problem. "Problem?" he says, like he thinks that's impossible, how could **he** have a problem. Yes, I told him, a problem, and here's why. We Americans say "stupid" when someone is ignorant or mentally challenged and we say "dumb" when we mean someone has poor judgment or makes a silly mistake. So, I said, Stephen—his name's Stephen—here's an example. When you decided we poor backward Yanks don't know the difference between the two words, that showed your ignorance about our language, so that was what we would call **stupid**. But you being **stupid** didn't stop there, I said. Oh no, instead of keeping your **stupid** idea to yourself, you opened your mouth to show us how **stupid** you really were. And that was what we call dumb, Stephen. Yep, that was **dumb**. (Laughs)

| Jane | (Smiles in spite of herself) How'd that go across? |
|------|----|

*It looks like Martin may have a pattern of starting the session with a prepared speech attacking someone: last time it was "women" and now "stupid Brits." This possible* SYMPTOMATIC ACT, *if it continues, would require Jane's therapeutic attention. In addition, it is the second example of an attack on someone with whom he has a social interaction: another defensive area of interest. Martin is obviously proud of himself for calling Stephen out, but Jane avoids taking a position on his anecdote and opts for seeking more information. If he's looking for praise from her that might suggest an early* TRANSFERENCE, *one where he sees her as a parental figure who can give praise or criticism and who must be impressed.*

| Martin | Everybody laughed, even the Brits. But not Stephen, of course. He sat there looking all glum and hurt. |
|------|----|

| Jane | And how did you feel? |
|------|----|

*She wants to focus on his emotional response, since he has so much difficulty acknowledging his feelings. This event parallels the one with Bettina: Martin again "teases" someone but does not appear to recognize the implicit hostility.*

| Martin | (Grins) Pretty good. |
|------|----|

| Jane | So, you didn't worry about what other people would think of you and you didn't just think the thoughts in your head. You spoke up. You were assertive. |
|------|----|

*With this statement Jane begins to lay a
FOUNDATION for a later opportunity to deal
with his COUNTERPHOBIC defense. Further,
Martin's answer ("Pretty good") shows
he's not aware of his emotions. He could
have identified, for example, his anger at the
patriotic insult, his contempt for the snooty
Brit, his joy at one-upping him, his pride at
scoring points with the rest of the group, and
so on. Jane puts into words for him that he
overcame his usual social anxiety and then she
REFRAMES his behavior as "assertive," rather
than the more negative label "aggressive."*

Martin.     (Smugly) Yeah, that's right. I felt pretty good.

Jane        Well, maybe we can figure out why this situation was
            different. What made you able to assert yourself with
            this group?

            *"Pretty good" seems to be all he can manage.
            Jane's suggestion is her attempt to use this
            incident to advance the TREATMENT PLAN.*

Martin      Yeah… Well, for one thing, these guys were just vis-
            iting. Tomorrow they head back to London.

Jane        So it was safer. You made Stephen look like a fool and
            there were no long-term consequences. By the way,
            were there any women around when you were at lunch?

            *She makes the issue of his feeling of safety
            overt by NAMING it, and then implies that he
            feels safer with men.*

Martin      Nope. Just the three of them, me, and two guys from
            my section. And I didn't make him look like a fool.
            He did that to himself. I just pointed it out.

| | |
|---|---|
| Jane | Do you think that made it easier for you to speak up? That they were all men. |

> *Jane wants to use this fresh data to continue the work from the previous session on how he relates to women. She ignores the other issue, his denial of his aggression and what it might mean: in his answer, he wasn't the attacker; the other man just made himself a victim.*

| | |
|---|---|
| Martin | Probably. But I didn't think about who was listening; I just said what I said. |

| | |
|---|---|
| Jane | Uh-huh. |

> *A neutral response that encourages him to continue.*

| | |
|---|---|
| Martin | I do better when I don't think about it too long first. It makes me self-conscious, and I worry how other people might react. |

| | |
|---|---|
| Jane | But in this case that didn't matter to you because you were never going to see those London people again. What does that tell you? |

> *She summarizes his reaction to help underline its importance.*

| | |
|---|---|
| Martin | (Frowns) It tells me it was a one-off. Not going to help me anywhere else. |

| | |
|---|---|
| Jane | In other words, you didn't care what they'd think of you. So, that raises the question of why other people's opinions are so important to you that you're usually not willing to risk saying what you feel. What do you think? |

*Jane is trying to make the most out of
this incident and is therefore being more
directive with her questions than she might
otherwise be.*

Martin      I think that's right.

Jane        Yes, but what makes you so sensitive to other peo-
            ple's opinions?

            *He gives a weak and limited response. She
            tries again.*

Martin      I don't know. (He's quiet for several moments, star-
            ing at the floor) Other people don't seem to care about
            that. They just say anything they feel like and if you
            don't like it, too bad. Me, it makes me cringe inside
            if I don't get a good reaction. I guess I'm just more
            sensitive to rejection.

                                          Time remaining
                                          35 minutes

Jane        Well, what makes you cringe? What do think it is
            about you that makes you more sensitive?

            *He responds with a better but still intellectual
            answer that is not very helpful. Jane keeps
            trying to have him look under the surface.*

Martin      (Shrugs) You tell me.

Jane        I'd like to hear your thoughts. You're the one with
            the feelings.

            *She reveals a little of her frustration, but
            sticks with the effort.*

Martin        Okay. I'll think about it. (He remains silent for a
              moment) I saw that lab tech again. Bettina.

Jane          Oh?

              *Instead of discussing his "thoughts," he
              offers a diversion, but to an important topic.
              Jane decides to go with it.*

Martin        Yeah. I ran into her on my way in this morning. We
              were heading for the elevator and I wasn't sure I
              should get in with her. So, I asked her to wait a min-
              ute and then I apologized. I said I was sorry I'd made
              her uncomfortable.

Jane          That's the word you used? Uncomfortable?

              *"Uncomfortable" sounds to Jane's ear like
              an intellectualized word.*

Martin        Actually I said I was sorry if I acted like a creep.

Jane          How'd she respond to that?

              *She could initiate a discussion on his word
              choice (picking a bland word rather than
              the more colorful one he actually used).
              Instead, she prompts him to continue with
              his account, since that seems to be the more
              important focus at this time.*

Martin        She just nodded and said thanks; then she went on to
              the elevator and I waited for the next one.

Jane          Is that what you expected?

*She wants to know what he imagined would happen; for example, if he thought his apology would reopen their troubled relationship.*

Martin   I didn't know what to expect. It wasn't something I planned to do. I saw her in the lobby and I just felt I should apologize, so I did.

Jane   Spur of the moment.

*Jane's comment is meant to identify this key behavioral maneuver. It is the second example in this session of Martin overcoming his social anxiety by acting on impulse (the first being his confrontation of the British visitor), suggesting that this behavior may be one of his coping skills. If so, it might be problematic: action without forethought could just as easily result in a bad outcome. A therapy* GOAL *is to overcome the anxiety through being less self-conscious.*

Martin   Yeah. I know I don't have a chance with her, so it wasn't me trying to start things up again. Not that there was anything much **to** start up.

Jane   Uhm-hmm.

*She makes a neutral sound to encourage him to continue.*

Martin   Women don't like me. I'm going to end up a creepy old bachelor, walking his dog twice a day and living alone till he dies.

Jane   That's quite a picture.

*Instead of further discussion of his problem
with Bettina he generalizes and exaggerates in
an attempt to use his* INTELLECTUAL DEFENSE
*against the pain of failing with her. Jane
could have challenged his diversion ("It's still
hard to talk about Bettina, isn't it?"), but she
doesn't quite recognize it in time and makes a
half-hearted* METACOMMUNICATION.

Martin   Yeah, my mother would have said I'm wallowing in self-pity again.

Jane   "Wallowing in self-pity"?

*Jane repeats his words to invite him to
elaborate.*

Martin   Yep. She didn't like to hear me say things like that.

Jane   Do you mean, she didn't want you to say how you were feeling?

*She invites him to explore the roots of his*
INTELLECTUAL DEFENSES.

Martin   Not exactly. That was more my father. "Suck it up," "Be a man."

Jane   Doesn't sound like either of them wanted to know what was going on with you.

*She tries to stay with the issue of his
intellectualizing.*

Martin   (Flatly) I guess not.

Jane   Do you think their attitude still affects you today?

*She tries again, this time with a more direct interpretation.*

Martin    Sometimes. Sometimes I can still hear them in my head.

Jane    Maybe they're in there even if you don't hear them.
*He has provided new information, suggesting his parents persist for him as INTROJECTED OBJECTS. She wants to build on it.*

Martin    You're right. They are. (His eyes fill with tears and he looks away)

Jane    What are you feeling right now?
*Martin has difficulty putting his feelings into words, so she asks a direct question.*

Martin    Sad. (He sniffs and wipes his eyes on his sleeve) Stupid, right?

Time remaining
25 minutes

Jane    Feelings aren't stupid.
*A statement rather than another question. She wants to both validate his feeling and help him accept being in touch with his emotional responses.*

Martin    I haven't lived at home since I left for college. I shouldn't let them influence me.

Jane    It's hard to ignore someone if they're living in your head.

*Another statement. He has incorporated his parents' repressive attitude. It seems to be one source of his inhibited emotions (but probably not the only one) and she tries to emphasize its importance to him.*

Martin        True. (Thinks for a moment) How do I get them out of there?

Jane          It helps knowing they're in there.

              *She prompts him to use this insight to resist the influence of his early training.*

Martin        Uh-huh.

Jane          Could you tell me more about your parents? What kind of people are they?

              *Martin's insight that his internalized parents exert some degree of critical oversight opens up a new area of investigation. Jane will need additional history to fully explore its influence.*

Martin        Busy. They're busy people. Always have been.

Jane          And what does that mean? Too busy for you?

              *She wants to maintain focus on how they have affected him.*

Martin        Exactly.

Jane          That seems the opposite of their being in your head.

              *Jane understands very well how apparently disinterested parents might still convey*

*their expectations and establish a set
of behavioral norms for their children.
Her comment invites Martin to maintain
concentration on their internalized
influence.*

Martin      Yeah. But they're never too busy to scrutinize my progress.

Jane      Are you saying they always find fault with you?

*She wants him to focus on the negative
influence that may contribute to his social
anxiety.*

Martin      Not always, but usually.

Jane      And that's how they were growing up, too?

*This question invites him to consider their
longstanding influence as a FOUNDATION for
connecting it to his present difficulties.*

Martin      Yep. "Be polite." "Don't make a scene." "Behave yourself."

Jane      Were you such a difficult child?

*Jane assumes he was a normal child, since
young children not yet fully socialized
normally act "impolite" or "make a
scene." Her question goes to Martin's self-
perception of his child-like behavior and
how his parents defined him. As such, it lays
a FOUNDATION to explore the topic.*

Martin      I guess I was. Difficult for them, anyway.

Jane          "Don't make a scene" sounds like you were brought
              up to be self-conscious.

                      *Now she can make a direct connection for
                      him between his parents' critique and his
                      adult sensitivity.*

Martin        (Nods) Right.

Jane          You think that's affected you to this day?

                      *His response ("Right") suggests he has
                      made an intellectual connection but not an
                      affective one.*

Martin        That sounds right.

Jane          You're father's a pharmacist?

                      *Same tentative answer. She decides to explore
                      his parents' treatment of his behavior as a
                      child by eliciting more about them.*

Martin        He is. That's the family business.

Jane          (Slightly puzzled) The **family** business?

Martin        My grandfather was a pharmacist. He was in World
              War II and then went back to school on the GI Bill.
              He had his own store. You know, an independent
              pharmacy. Don't know if those even exist any-
              more. Then, my father became a pharmacist, too,
              and he worked for his father in the store until the
              old man retired. He ran it for almost 20 years and
              then he sold out to Walgreens. That's the story,
              anyway.

Jane          The story? You don't believe it?

*He has recited the "family legend" but
seems skeptical. That may present an early
opening for him to reject his parents'
imposed self-consciousness.*

Martin    No, I do. It's just that he never liked being a pharmacist. I think he was glad to give it up. He retired after a few years working there as an employee.

Jane    If being a pharmacist was the family business, were you expected to go that route too?

*In other words: did he disappoint them with
his career choice?*

Martin    (Chuckles) I could've, sure. Luckily, I won a science fair competition in high school. It got me some scholarship money and I went for a biochem degree. Otherwise I'd probably be filling scrips behind a counter somewhere.

Jane    How'd your father feel about that?

*If it was a source of disapproval, Jane wants
him to confront it.*

Martin    He was okay with it.

*Time remaining
15 minutes*

Jane    And your mother? What's she like?

*The discussion about his father did not elicit
much emotion. "Okay with it" doesn't sound
like his father was overtly proud of him. She
decides to switch to his mother.*

Martin          Well, like I told you, she taught first and second grade. I think she still treats me like I'm seven. (Laughs) She's still my mommy.

Jane             And is that good or bad?

*She probes whether his "mommy" in his head is a critical or supportive internalized voice.*

Martin          (Shrugs) A little of both, I suppose.

Jane             So, when you said before that they're in your head, is it more your Mommy in there or your father?

*Martin has not been able to discuss the emotional side of his parents' influence. Jane tries to bring the focus back to the original topic. She sticks with his word, Mommy, to match his DICTION.*

Martin          (Pauses with a thoughtful expression) More my father. You know, he didn't marry my mother until he was 40. And when I came along he was 46. I don't think he expected to have any children.

Jane             You weren't a planned pregnancy?

*Martin uses the question of his conception to divert from the issue of his father's critical voice. Jane misses the diversion.*

Martin          (Shakes his head) I think I was an accident.

Jane             An accident.

*She echoes the word to emphasize its possible emotional impact.*

Martin          They never said that. That's just my idea.

| Jane | So, your parents didn't want you, they were critical of your behavior growing up— |
| --- | --- |
| | *She recognizes the diversion and uses it to return to topic.* |

| Martin | They still are. |
| --- | --- |

| Jane | —and now they're in your head. |
| --- | --- |
| | *Jane returns to the exact wording of the earlier discussion to further focus on it.* |

| Martin | Doesn't sound too good. (Pauses) Hey, I've got a joke to tell you. What's the best thing about 27 year old virgins? |
| --- | --- |

| Jane | (Says nothing. Waits, with neutral expression.) |
| --- | --- |
| | *This sudden digression suggests that the topic of his parent's disapproval has become too painful to pursue. Surprised at the abrupt change, Jane isn't sure what to say about this obvious defensive effort.* |

| Martin | OK. The best thing about 27 year old virgins is that there are 20 of them! (When Jane doesn't react) What? You don't think that's funny? |
| --- | --- |

| Jane | (Shrugs) I get it, but I'm curious that you want to change the subject with a pedophilia joke. |
| --- | --- |
| | *She labels the joke with a term that has a negative connotation. Her punitive choice reflects her disappointment that he chose to stop what seemed a useful discussion, but a less pejorative label would have been better for the THERAPEUTIC ALLIANCE. She risks* |

*sounding like his censorious parents. Although Jane avoids a direct "why" question by this construction, she still can identify his change of subject as a problem. There's no evidence from earlier sessions that Martin has sexual feelings toward children—although the absence of evidence isn't evidence of absence—but this inappropriate joke is consistent with his social awkwardness and "tin ear" about how others, especially women, may perceive him.*

Martin        Pedophilia? Hey, it's a joke. That's all. I don't have a thing for little girls.

Jane          (In a neutral tone) OK.

*As usual, he's surprised that someone else doesn't see things the way he does. She recognizes she has erred in using such a harsh word, but doesn't see how she can back off without causing more problems.*

Martin        I don't! (Frowns) Jeeze. You shrinks!

Jane          What about us shrinks?

*Jane could let Martin's exasperated remark pass, but she wants to respond to any hint of negative TRANSFERENCE, as flagged by the use of the derogatory term "shrink." In this case, the idea that Jane can't take a joke because of her role as his therapist might indicate that Martin wants to have a more personal relationship, one outside the formal therapist–patient dyad, and a potential BOUNDARY VIOLATION.*

Martin     (Shakes his head with a can-you-believe-this expression) Nothing. Never mind. (He falls silent. Several minutes pass.)

Jane     Do you suppose you told that joke because you wanted to change the subject?

> *She has to decide how to handle his silence, a kind of* RESISTANCE, *because the* THERAPEUTIC ALLIANCE *has been stressed by her refusal to be diverted by his inappropriate joke. She could wait it out. She could try a* METACOMMUNICATION *("Are you sulking?"). She could flag his anger picking up on his calling her a shrink. At this early stage of therapy, however, these more stressful* TACTICS *might weaken the alliance further, so she opts for a different* METACOMMUNICATION *and the more neutral response of simply asking another question.*

Martin     No, no. The joke just popped into my mind and I thought you'd laugh.

Jane     So it was like what happened at lunch today with those British visitors. You spoke without thinking and you weren't self-conscious.

> *She links the two incidents to emphasize her interpretation that his spontaneous or impulsive interactions, that don't give him time to worry about the consequences, are his only way of overcoming his social anxiety. A* COUNTERPHOBIC *defense mechanism.*

Martin     (Grumbling) Yeah. I guess so.

Jane            But in this case, you didn't get the reaction you expected.

*He offers a grudging agreement. He is still*
*sulking about her reaction to his joke. A*
*METACOMMUNICATION about his surly mood*
*might now be better than her persistence on*
*her INTERPRETATION, but the session is almost*
*over, and time may not allow for a useful*
*discussion.*

Martin          (Low voice) No.

Jane            So I was thinking about something you do that maybe
                is a pattern for you. You remember last time you made
                that speech about what devious snakes and fortune
                hunters women were and today you started off with
                that anecdote about putting that British visitor in his
                place. And then, just now, we're talking about some
                painful things from your childhood and you pop up
                with a joke about little girls.

Martin          So what, I'm shooting my mouth off too much? I
                should keep my ideas to myself?

Jane            Isn't that the opposite of what we're trying to do?

*She uses a question to rebut his obvious*
*misstatement, a kind of aggressive RESISTANCE.*

Martin          I would have thought so, but then what are you trying
                to tell me?

                                                    Time remaining
                                                    5 minutes

Jane            Do you see anything in common about those three
                examples I just mentioned?

*She tries again to get his cooperation in
looking at his behavior.*

Martin          Sure. You think I'm a jerk who can't keep his mouth
                shut.

Jane            That's one way to look at it, I guess. I had a different
                thought. I think maybe it's a technique you use to
                help yourself get over your shyness and your worry
                about people judging you.

                *Her interest in offering this
                INTERPRETATION makes her ignore
                his self-critical comment.*

Martin          (Puzzled) …What?

Jane            Let's say you're standing outside of a room. You know
                you want to go in there but you're not sure it's safe. You
                can't bring yourself to just calmly walk in because you
                think it may be dangerous. So, what do you do? You put
                your fists up and you rush in as fast as you can before
                you can think about what you're risking. Just plunge
                right in, ready for a fight, and hope for the best.

                *Given his apparent confusion about her
                INTERPRETATION, she chooses a RHETORICAL
                approach using a metaphor to describe his
                COUNTERPHOBIC defense.*

Martin          That's what I do when I tell people things they don't
                want to hear?

Jane            What do you think?

                *He seems unusually dense about this
                INTERPRETATION, suggesting his confusion*

*is a defensive effort to reject her idea. The strength of his reaction against it implies it is on target but will need further discussion to WORK IT THROUGH.*

Martin        Yeah, maybe. I'll have to think about that some more.

Jane          Speaking without thinking means you don't let yourself worry about how it's going to come across, how other people are going to think about you. Whether you'll be accepted or make a fool of yourself.

              *Her repetition of her point may be somewhat heavy-handed, given his sullen behavior.*

Martin        (Irritated) Sounds like I'm damned if I do and damned if I don't.

Jane          Or, maybe the problem isn't whether **you** think first or not but it's whether you need to worry so much about what **other** people might think.

              *Again, she ignores his attitude and emphasizes her point.*

Martin        That's what you think?

Jane          It's worth considering.

              *Meaning, we should talk more about this topic.*

Martin        Okay.

Jane          Our time is up for today and we have to stop.

              *The termination formula indicates no more discussion for today.*

Martin        (Shakes his head slowly, then gets up and leaves without another word)

### Discussion

The eagerness with which Martin awaited the beginning of this session, when he could relate his "victory" over the condescending British visitor, reflects how empty his life is. He has no one to share his success with except his therapist. His reliance on the therapy relationship may become a problem, especially in the termination phase of his treatment.

The influence of his previous and unsuccessful therapy with the psychoanalyst—a silent, passive, out of sight figure—has led Jane to take a more active role. Partly, this approach is an educational attempt to introduce him to the more engaged activity of psychotherapy and partly it reflects her frustration with the poorly focused and discursive style Martin has learned in his four years of treatment. She wants him to be more actively engaged in a process that will lead to success in reaching their therapy goals.

For the second time Martin comes in with a "prepared statement," a story of triumph over a British visitor who insults American speech. In both recitations he presents himself as justifiably outraged at being looked down upon, first by predatory women and then by snooty foreigners.

Jane recognizes these outbursts as "set pieces," probably conceived and crafted by Martin ahead of his appointment. Various hypotheses suggest themselves to her to explain this unusual behavior. It could be he wants to show he is in control of the agenda. Perhaps he wants to impress her with his superior intellect. Or does he believe he must bring in some interesting new material to attract her interest and justify his taking up her time? Maybe he thinks she will be more helpful to him if he demonstrates how effectively he analyzes situations on his own: sort of a fellow therapist. Does he run down the therapy clock so there is less time to scrutinize his inner thoughts and problems?

Any or all of these hypotheses might turn out to true, but at this early stage of therapy Jane does not have enough evidence to judge any of them. When the third instance occurs, however, and Martin interrupts an important discussion of his parents' influence on him with an inappropriate joke about sexual abuse of children, Jane feels she must address it, even with only a limited understanding of its significance.

The session ends with Martin still angry with her, ostensibly because she failed to appreciate his joke with its clever word play about seven year old virgins, but perhaps also or more significantly because she exposed his "weakness" in the discussion about his sensitivity to rejection, the core of his social anxiety. His attempt to divert her with the joke failed and his frustration led to his anger. The strain on the therapeutic alliance could become a threat to the therapy. At worst, for example, he could cancel the next session or even drop out of treatment. A more likely result would be his arriving late to the next session and even subsequent sessions. His acting out behavior would then require Jane to take time away from their treatment goals to deal with the threat, since if Martin is not in the office or truncates the therapy time by his lateness, that will pose a threat to his treatment.

## Notes

1  A transactional formulation might also be considered because so much of his day-to-day difficulties involve interactions with other people. This narrower category would dictate a less useful treatment plan.
2  A patient switching from one type of therapy to another often requires some period of "retraining" before the new approach can be successful.

## Reference

Erikson, E. H. (1959). Identity and the life cycle: Selected papers. *Psychological Issues*, 1, 1–171.

# Dave

## A Serial Adulterer

## Referral

Dave is self-referred after finding Jane's private practice through an internet search. He called the office and requested an appointment, saying "I want to save my marriage."

## Preparation

Jane sometimes receives background material from another provider or others involved in the referral. She looks over anything sent, but she does not seek outside information, for example by doing an online search, because she doesn't want to be influenced before she can form her own impressions. In this case, where Dave is self-referred, she has no information.

Jane tries to approach each client with an open mind. When she sees a potential new client, in addition to the regular history and mental status material, Jane always looks for the answers to three questions:

1.  Why did this person come *here*?

    Other alternatives for help with behavioral problems include family physicians, friends, mentors, family members, life coaches, pastoral counselors, and even the plethora of self-help books. One early study found that nearly three-quarters of people with a diagnosable behavioral disorder did **not** seek professional help of any kind (Regier et al., 1993) and that only half of the remaining one-quarter went to a behavioral health provider (Narrow et al., 1993). Yet Jane's new client has chosen her, a psychotherapist, with all its

DOI: 10.4324/9781003353003-10

potential social stigma, expense and time commitment. She wants to know why she was selected: what expectations, biases and hidden agenda influenced this choice.

2.  Why did this person come *now*?

Most behavioral problems are longstanding and tolerated, even if it means drastic changes or restrictions in lifestyle or social activity. At some point in time a change occurs in this homeostatic system and precipitates the seeking of outside help. Jane wants to know what that precipitant was.

3.  What does this person *want*?

This question is always the most important because it will influence the choice of treatment. Sometimes the new person can state clearly what outcome they want to achieve through psychotherapy, but other, less appropriate goals may be present.[1] Jane tries to clarify what the person wants in their initial meeting, but sometimes the true request does not emerge until later in the therapy. The treatment contract must then be renegotiated or at least modified to reflect this change.

## SESSION ONE

Dave arrives on time and is reading on his phone when Jane opens the door to her office. He is a trim man of medium height. His dark hair is brushed straight back from his forehead. He wears a plaid sports coat and dark slacks. His shoes are polished to a high shine. He has a large "pinky ring" set with a black stone on his left hand but no wedding ring. He enters the office with a bounce in his step and drops into his chair. He appears relaxed and confident.

Jane takes her seat. She usually begins by asking, "What can I do for you?"[2] Dave, however, doesn't wait for her to speak.

Time remaining
45 minutes

Dave          (Looking around the room) Hey, nice office. I always wondered what this would be like. You don't have a couch.

| | |
|---|---|
| Jane | No, that's right. No couch. |

*Jane answers him simply, without explaining why she does not offer him (or anyone) classical psychoanalysis. She regards this question as the indirect beginning of the negotiation toward a TREATMENT CONTRACT. Dave is trying to establish the parameters of the encounter, although it is doubtful he is aware of it.*

| | |
|---|---|
| Dave | And aren't you supposed to have a pad and pen to take notes? |
| Jane | I don't take notes while we're talking. I do keep a record of our sessions and make notes afterward. |

*These questions reveal Dave's rather naïve understanding of therapy. Jane accepts his questions as an attempt to better define her role. Like the psychoanalytic couch, this is another popular image. TV and film therapists are almost always identified using a pen and notebook, the way doctors and nurses wear a stethoscope or construction workers a hard hat.[3] She gives a similar short explanation, rather than discussing how these stereotypes might influence their work together. Jane lets him know that she does keep a record of what he tells her, since this issue may also be part of the TREATMENT CONTRACT.*

| | |
|---|---|
| Dave | Okay, so what's the plan here? |
| Jane | The idea is for us to focus on your problems and see how you can change. |

*She offers a vague educational statement to emphasize that his behavior will be*

*the focus of their work together. Again,*
*Dave's question is helpful in establishing a*
TREATMENT CONTRACT.

Dave    Right. Well, my main problem right now is my wife is pissed, really pissed, because she found out that I was seeing someone else. Another woman. (Grins) But I want to be completely honest here: what she doesn't know is that she wasn't the first.

Jane    No?

*She's not surprised to hear this, but makes*
*a neutral inquiry to encourage him to*
*elaborate. His use of the phrase, "I want to*
*be completely honest," makes Jane wonder*
*why he needs to reassure her. So far, she has*
*the answer to one question: why now? The*
*precipitant is that his wife learned about his*
*infidelity.*

Dave    No. I've had other hook-ups. More than a few, to be honest, that she doesn't know about, and if she ever finds out... (Looks around) You're not recording this, right? Isn't everything I tell you confidential? I mean, you could never tell her.

Jane    Everything we discuss is confidential. I wouldn't disclose anything we talk about here unless you asked me to. We have what's called a limited privilege. That means there are two exceptions. If I was ordered by a court is one and the other is if you tell me you plan to physically hurt someone. That's called a duty to warn[4] and I would have to do what I could to prevent that.

*Jane notes his word, "hook-ups," a term for*
*casual sex more appropriate for an unmarried*

*man in the dating scene. She now has at least
part of the answer to her second question: why
here? He wants to maintain the confidentiality
she offers as a behavioral health professional,
a protection he might not be able to get with
other sources of help. So, his question about
note-taking wasn't just simple curiosity. She
wants to reassure him but also to be clear
about the* BOUNDARIES. *It's important for Dave
to understand that therapists are not quite as
protected as lawyers and clergy. Although
Dave's question was only about his wife,
she uses the opportunity to clearly define the
limitations of the privilege. Also, she notes he
has mentioned being "honest" twice in a row
and Jane wonders if honesty is a problem for
him. So far, Dave has controlled the interview
with his questions, a reversal of the usual
relationship. Jane senses he wants to establish
his dominance and wonders if that's why he
chose a female therapist.*

Dave    I'm not going to attack anybody. (Grins) You know,
make love not war, that's where I'm at.

Jane    (Nods) So, you were saying…

*Jane begins to feel that his frequent grinning
is an insincere habit, perhaps part of his
sales approach. She chooses to steer him
back to the topic rather than to have a more
theoretical discussion.*

Dave    Yeah. It's just that there've been other women, that
my wife doesn't know about. (A microexpression
appears: perhaps anxiety, perhaps disgust)

| | |
|---|---|
| Jane | And your wife's name is…? |
| | *Jane notices the fleeting change in his expression but does not consciously identify it, even though it makes her feel uneasy. Jane senses that Dave wants to discuss his problem in the abstract, so she wants to emphasize the reality of his wife's existence.* |
| Dave | Marie. |
| Jane | And how long are you and Marie married? |
| | *Jane begins to take back some control of the interview.* |
| Dave | Twelve years. Thirteen next month. |
| Jane | What's Marie like? |
| | *She repeats the name to underline the reality of the woman.* |
| Dave | (Thoughtfully) What is she like… She's very social, athletic. She plays tennis. She's a great mom. She works part-time as a medical assistant for a dermatology practice. |
| Jane | Can you tell me a little more about yourself? How old are you? What do you do? What's your background like? |
| | *Everything he says about Marie is impersonal. Nothing about what she's like as a person. It's too soon to confront him with that so she asks for more information about him.* |

| Dave | Sure. I'm 40. We have two kids. Two girls. They're 10 and 7. I'm in Real Estate. I'm a broker, residential sales. |

| Jane | What about your family growing up? |

*Again, he mentions his children but not their names. Jane is beginning to sense a problem with Dave's relationships with other people. Since this is an initial interview, Jane moves on to get additional history.*

| Dave | Yeah. My mother died when I was seven and a few years later my dad married a woman with two kids of her own. I was ten and she had a daughter nine and a son who was five at the time, so, you know, instant family. (Grins) |

| Jane | That sounds like a pretty rough period of your life. |

*She offers a* METACOMMUNICATION *to see if he will tell her any of the emotional consequences.*

| Dave | Yeah. Wasn't good, but my stepmother turned out okay. |

Time remaining
35 minutes

| Jane | How far did you go in school? |

*Losing his mother at seven must have been a disaster for him, but Dave mentions it without affect. With a different client, Jane might have focused on this trauma. Again, he mentions the family members by role rather than by name. Although this pattern is not dispositive, she nevertheless forms a*

> *tentative HYPOTHESIS that Dave sees other people as objects to use or discard. If true, it suggests he might have SOCIOPATHIC traits and is not a good therapy candidate.*

Dave
High school and a couple years of college. High school was great. I ran track, played basketball. I was on the football team. Best years of my life, really. (Grimaces) It's been downhill ever since.

Jane
You sound discouraged. Any problems with depression? Ever feel suicidal?

> *She takes advantage of this opening to ask a required safety question.*

Dave
(With raised eyebrows) Christ, no!

Jane
But "downhill ever since."

> *Having ascertained he isn't at risk, she needs to bring him back to the history.*

Dave
Yep. (Stares off for a moment) So I tried college but it wasn't working out and I needed to start earning a living, so I quit and took the broker course, got my license and here I am.

Jane
And how long have you been seeing other women?

> *Jane is tempted to explore his college failure but decides to continue with his present difficulties. She wants to define the extent of the infidelity. She also contemplates the HYPOTHESIS that his pursuit of other women might reflect his idealizing of his high school years and his wish to continue his remembered former success. If so,*

*this self-image would suggest a failure of
adult development, the transition from a
young adult seeking a partner to a stable
relationship in a new family.*

Dave      Quite a while. Almost from the beginning. I'm not
proud of it. It's not something I'd planned to do, but
opportunities present themselves and I can't help taking advantage of them. (Grins)

Jane      Opportunities? How many other women have there
been?

*Concrete details will help to anchor the
reality of his behavior. His statement that
"he can't help taking advantage" suggests
he views his promiscuity as outside of his
control. This concept might prove a serious
challenge to the therapy. And why, she
wonders, does he keep grinning?*

Dave      Not sure. I guess somewhere between a dozen and
two dozen. Why?

Jane      It sounds like you almost always have another sexual
partner.

*Jane has the impression from the way he
discusses his behavior that the other women
are simply useful and not people he has any
personal feelings about. She chooses the
term, "sexual partner," a deliberate change
of* DICTION, *using a more "clinical" term, to
further define his treatment of them.*

Dave      Yeah. It's like that song. (Sings) "When I'm not near
the girl I love, I love the girl I'm near."

Jane            (Nods)

*Jane recognizes the tune from an old
musical, Finian's Rainbow, sung by an
amorous leprechaun. Later in therapy
she might be able to use this reference to
discuss his responsibility for his behavior.
At this early stage, however, it would be
premature, since she has not completed a
FORMULATION or established a TREATMENT
PLAN, so she simply files it away.*

Dave            Selling real estate's not an office job, you know.
                I'm always out and about. I meet a lot of people and
                sometimes that means women looking for a hook-up.

Jane            You're saying it's the women who initiate these
                relationships?

                *Jane wants to challenge his implication that
                he's not responsible for this behavior and
                therefore unable to change it.*

Dave            Well, mostly. I mean, I'm alert to the possibilities.
                (Broad smile) But, seriously, there are women out
                there, and I mean lots of them, who are just looking
                for somebody new. Maybe they're bored with who-
                ever they're with or they just like sex or I don't know
                what all the reasons are. (Shakes his head) So whether
                I make the first move or they do, they're interested.
                And you know, they'll do anything you want when
                they're auditioning.

Jane            Auditioning?

                *An unusual word. Jane wants to know what
                he means.*

| Dave | Yeah. You know, when they think they might have a future with you, maybe even get married, and they're willing to go along with whatever you suggest. Like, you say, let's go to the opera and they'll say sure I love opera when the truth is they wouldn't be caught dead in an opera. By the way, are you married? |
|---|---|
| Jane | You're curious about me. |
| | *Jane responds to the BOUNDARY VIOLATION with a METACOMMUNICATION instead of an answer to his question. She wonders whether he's coming on to her. Does he see her as a professional or just another potential conquest? She might need to address this problem at a later time if other instances appear, but for now she wants to continue the assessment.* |
| Dave | Yeah, just wondering if you have any real experience in this area, but never mind… The point is I'm a normal guy and if I see some girl who's attractive and available, what am I going to do? (Pauses) But I'm not saying I have nothing to do with it. |
| Jane | Well, that's hopeful. |
| | *She dangles the comment, inviting him to ask what she means. Again he suggests a "normal guy" would act the way he does, as if his infidelity is not a real problem.* |
| Dave | What do you mean? |
| Jane | If you had nothing to do with it we wouldn't have any way for the therapy to help you. The idea here is for you to change. |

*An important question Jane needs to answer is
her third: what does he want? Is his motivation
for therapy a manipulation to pacify his angry
wife or is he motivated to change the behavior
that caused his current problems? She
emphasizes that behavior change is the AIM
of their work together, not, as she suspects,
merely appeasing his angry wife.*

Dave        That might be tough. You know, the spirit is willing
            but the flesh is weak.

                                            Time remaining
                                            25 minutes

Jane        You're quoting the bible?[5]

            *He implies that he is unable to control
            his behavior. Jane could reemphasize her
            previous statement, but instead simply
            implies that it's not a biblical problem. Her
            relatively neutral response might be a lost
            opportunity to discuss his responsibility for
            his philandering.*

Dave        Am I? (Grins) Well, there's a lot of wisdom in the
            good book.

Jane        Yes, but you were saying this is a longstanding…
            pattern of yours. Can you say more about that?

            *Again, she passes up a discussion of
            responsibility in favor of gathering more
            information.*

Dave        Sure. (He stares out the window for a moment) So,
            I've met a lot of women over the years. Selling and
            just being out and about, and it's like I said: some of

them have shown an interest. And when they do, I can't resist. (Shrugs and looks pleased)

Jane   Anybody in particular? Someone you had a longer-term relationship with?

> *Testing her HYPOTHESIS, she asks if any of his sexual partners were more than an outlet for him. He evidently gets a narcissistic boost from the idea that women find him desirable, another possible roadblock to a possible behavior change.*

Dave   Yeah, a couple. And, of course, the latest one. That's how my wife found out about it. The bitch called my house.

Jane   Let's talk about that one then. What's the bitch's name? How long were you seeing her?

> *She mirrors his DICTION, repeating the word, "bitch." Again, she wonders whether he sees the woman as a real person.*

Dave   Peggy. She was looking at properties because she was moving here for work. She has one of those tech jobs. She's single. We started by having drinks—so we could, you know (uses finger quotes), "discuss her move"—and then dinner and one thing led to another.

Jane   And how long ago was this?

> *Asking for more information but also laying a FOUNDATION for her HYPOTHESIS.*

Dave   Oh, about six months.

Jane                Did Peggy know you were married?

*She uses the woman's name to see if he can*
*be more personal in the discussion: not "that*
*bitch" or "she."*

Dave                (Shakes his head) Not at first. I didn't mention it and
she didn't ask. I guess she just assumed I was avail-
able. (He holds up his left hand) As you can see, I
don't wear a ring. It was when it did come out, that
I was married, that the trouble started. She must
have thought we had (he again makes air quotes
with his fingers) "a relationship," that it would go
somewhere. To me, it was always just sex. (Shakes
his head) Women! Always looking for more.

Jane                Are you saying you had no part in the misunderstanding? That it was all Peggy and what **she** wanted and
you were just an innocent participant? Doesn't that
sound suspicious to you?

*She begins to challenge his version of the*
*events.*

Dave                (Crosses his arms) Well, okay, if you put it that way,
sure. I didn't tell her because, you know, I didn't
want to screw things up. But she didn't ask, at first,
and when it did come up—I'm not sure, to tell you
the truth, why it did. (Frowns) But when it did I was
honest about it. I told her I was married. (Pauses)
Well, truth to tell, it was more than honesty. I didn't
want her to get any ideas that I was available.

Jane                How'd Peggy take the news?

*Again she notes his use of the phrases "to*
*tell you the truth" and "truth to tell" and*
*being "honest" while actually revealing*

*that he has been neither truthful nor honest in these relationships. At this point Jane becomes aware of a growing dislike for this man that could be a barrier to their work together.*

Dave    (Holds out his hands, palms up) What can I say? She was **not** happy. She went apeshit. That was her first reaction. She threw a fork at me. Luckily she missed (giggles) and then she wanted to know when I was going to get a divorce. Not if... when. So I had to explain I was never going to leave my kids, so no divorce.

Jane    The reason was the kids? Not Marie?

*She confronts him with the idea (not yet directly expressed) that his relationship with Marie is deeply flawed.*

Dave    No, I thought I'd better leave Marie out of it. (Shakes his head) No telling what she'd throw next.

Jane    What do you think Peggy was feeling during this discussion?

*He sees Peggy's upset as a problem to be managed, while he appears to deny any harm he has done her. Jane tries to focus him on Peggy, but again she is aware of her antipathy to his callous behavior.*

Dave    Feeling?

Jane    Yes. You're talking about what she did. What do you think were her emotions on hearing this news from you?

*She tries to make explicit his unawareness*
*of Peggy as a person, partly in exasperation*
*and partly to test her* HYPOTHESIS.

Dave        (Shrugs) Well, obviously, she was pissed.

Jane        And why was she pissed, do you think?

*She echoes his word, "pissed," to continue*
*to match his* DICTION. *She tries again to*
*focus him on Peggy's feelings. She might*
*have suggested other emotions that Dave*
*is missing—such as dismay, shame, regret,*
*chagrin, embarrassment, disappointment,*
*shock, anxiety—none of which he seems*
*capable of recognizing. At this point she*
*concludes that his indifference reflects a*
SOCIOPATHIC PERSONALITY.

Dave        I don't get your question. She thought we were
            heading toward marriage and then she finds out
            we're not. So, she's pissed. She's not getting what
            she wants.

                                            Time remaining
                                            15 minutes

Jane        Let's see if I've got the right picture here. You were
            seeing Peggy for six months. You never told her you
            were married with two kids. When she found out,
            Peggy was angry and that's it?

*Jane tries to confront him with his*
*problematic behavior by summarizing*
*it for him.*

Dave        Yeah.

| | |
|---|---|
| Jane | Huh! |

*Jane's not sure what to say next and makes a non-committal sound. She is unable to form a useful HYPOTHESIS about his behavior. Could it be related to losing his mother at an early age? Is it simply lust? Does he have power issues, with each "conquest" a trophy? So far, she lacks the data to say.*

| | |
|---|---|
| Dave | What? |

| | |
|---|---|
| Jane | What attracted you to Peggy in the first place? |

*She decides to get more history about the current problem.*

| | |
|---|---|
| Dave | (Grins) She's good looking and she was available? |

| | |
|---|---|
| Jane | But you kept seeing her. Longer than you usually did. |

*She prompts him to say more about it.*

| | |
|---|---|
| Dave | Like I said, she was attractive and available. Maybe that was my mistake. Usually, it's one and done. I shouldn't have kept on seeing her. |

| | |
|---|---|
| Jane | But what was she like as a person? |

*Jane says this with a touch of irritation that she recognizes as her negative feeling about him.*

| | |
|---|---|
| Dave | (Frowns) As a person. She was smart. Had a good sense of humor. The sex was good… Not sure what you're getting at here. |

Jane    I guess what I'm sensing here is that Peggy was more important to you for her external characteristics, her physical attractiveness, rather than for what kind of person she was.

> *She decides to spell it out for him to see whether he can recognize the problem with his predatory behavior.*

Dave    Yeah, well sure. That's true.

Jane    And how about Marie? What kind of person is she?

> *So if Peggy is only a sexual object for him, what about his wife? Jane makes a semi-judgmental statement that reflects her potential alliance with his wife. Again, not a helpful response to Dave, since he is the one she should be forming a WORKING ALLIANCE with.*

Dave    Marie? She's steady. A good mother. A good cook. Not great in bed, but, what the hell, after you've been married awhile, that happens. She's good at her job, brings in a steady income. Real estate, you know, has its ups and downs. Sometimes the market's hot, sometimes it's not. So it's good we can count on her paycheck.

Jane    So Marie is useful? She keeps the house running and brings in a paycheck?

> *He defines Marie by his perception of her as a series of functions: homemaker, second income earner.*

Dave    (Warily) You could put it like that.

| Jane | And no big problems at work? |
|------|------|

> *Laying a FOUNDATION for other sources of his behavior, such as stress at work.*

| Dave | No. Not at the moment, anyway. People are buying bigger and better homes than they need. I read where that's called the commodity self. People define themselves by what they own. So that's good for me. High-priced homes mean bigger commissions. |
|------|------|

| Jane | Uh huh. And how are the kids doing? |
|------|------|

> *Jane wonders if his reference to socioeconomic theory is an attempt to impress her. The other implication is the way he sees his potential buyers as financial opportunities rather than as people he could help, consistent with his attitude toward women as sexual objects. She continues to ask about other problem areas in his life.*

| Dave | They're great. Why are you asking all this? |
|------|------|

| Jane | Just wondering if you seeing other women is a result of stresses elsewhere. |
|------|------|

> *As part of the FOUNDATION she wants to evaluate other influences on his relationships with other women.*

| Dave | (Nods his understanding) I'd say not. |
|------|------|

| Jane | So, what do you think is the reason behind all your... extramarital activities? |
|------|------|

> *Jane chooses a neutral term for his adultery to make her question as unbiased as*

*possible. She wonders if he can provide any insight into his behavior.*

Dave    Why do I do it? (Frowns, as if thinking) It's like that old saying. Why does a dog lick its balls? Because it can. (Smiles)

Jane    That's it? Opportunity knocks and you answer?

*She tries to confront him.*

Dave    Right.

Jane    In other words, you're not actively looking yourself, but when women show an interest you seize the chance.

*She makes an overt statement to see if there's more to it.*

Dave    I guess so. Although, to be honest, I'm not exactly **not** looking, myself.

Jane    Uh-huh.

*Apparently there are no other influences. He is a sexual opportunist with no guilt about his activities. Jane realizes there is little here to work with, no reasonable basis for therapy.*

Dave    I'm not seeing anyone now.

Jane    Too risky?

*Jane feels more certain that he is, technically speaking, a sociopath, and kind of a sleaze. He is concealing his adultery because he needs to control his wife's reaction to finding out about Peggy. He has no remorse about*

*having hurt her or about his treatment of the
other woman. She doesn't like him and she
realizes he has a limited idea about therapy.*

Dave            That's part of it.

Jane            And the other part…?

*Jane doesn't think he has another reason,
but asks anyway.*

Dave            Well, that's why I'm here. I need to reassess this. I
think I've got a handle on it for now. She thinks it
was a one-off, a slip. She's naturally a forgiving person, but if it happens again, and Marie finds out, it's
going to be a massive problem.

Jane            But if Marie didn't find out, you'd be all right with it?

*So, he's stated "what he wants." He wants
a reliable shield against any damage to
his marriage if more information about his
infidelity, past and probably future, reaches
Marie. The danger is that he could face a
divorce with the loss of Marie's income and,
perhaps, his contact with his children. This is
a critical issue: can therapy help him change?
Is he motivated to change? Does he have any
moral or ethical qualms about his behavior
that might fuel an effort to modify it?*

Dave            I guess that's true. I mean, what can I say? It's not
like I don't enjoy myself. But it's risk/benefit. I don't
want to mess up my family but, if I'm completely
honest about it, I can't say I want to stop. My mistake was I kept seeing Peggy and she got ideas on her

own. So maybe that's the answer. One night stands and then that's it.

Time remaining
5 minutes

Jane  So the problem isn't what you're doing. It's whether you can get away with it?

> *Again, it sounds like what he wants is a better way to disguise his serial adultery so Marie doesn't make his life unpleasant. He can tell her he's "in therapy" and working on his "problem." Jane wants no part of a treatment contract based on aiding and abetting him in this effort. She hopes that's not all it is and restates his response in order to give him one last opportunity to modify it.*

Dave  (Shrugs) I know it doesn't sound so good but I've got to be honest about it.

Jane  (Frowns) I see.

> *Jane has reached a decision: she will not continue with this man. Unfortunately, the session is near its end and she realizes that rejecting him will be a disappointment with too little time left to WORK IT THROUGH with him. She is unwilling, however, to schedule another visit for that purpose.*

Dave  You don't sound happy about it.

Jane  It's not whether I'm happy. It's a question of whether therapy is the way to go.

> *Instead of trying for a* THERAPEUTIC
> CONTRACT, *Jane now has to disengage as
> smoothly as possible.*

Dave      That's why I'm here.

Jane      Psychotherapy can't help everybody. I'm not sure we have a basis to proceed.

> *She starts out with a general statement, hoping
> to soften the rejection.*

Dave      What are you saying?

Jane      I don't think I can help you with this problem.

> *And then makes it specific. She makes herself
> the focus and avoids listing what it is about
> him and thus blaming him, not wanting to
> provoke an argument at this late stage of the
> session.*

Dave      You don't?

Jane      No. I'm sorry, but I don't think I should see you again.

> *She wants to be clear that she is not offering
> him any treatment and that there is no
> ambiguity about her decision.*

Dave      You're throwing me out? Unbelievable. (Stares at her) So what should I do now?

Jane      That's up to you. If you want to try with someone else, I can give you the names of other therapists. They may feel differently about it.

> *This offer is more a medicolegal statement to show she isn't abandoning him. She will also send him a letter confirming her decision and renewing her offer to make a referral.*

Dave    (Scowls) Thanks for nothing! I've just been wasting my time here. I don't need to go anywhere else. I'll just have to figure it out on my own.

Jane    Well, it's up to you. But our time is up and we have to stop.

> *Jane regrets having to deliver a narcissistic blow to this man and she feels disappointed that the encounter ends this way, but she is clear in her own mind that therapy would be unsuccessful and used by Dave only to manipulate his wife.*

Dave    (Sits for a moment, his expression angry, and then he storms out)

Jane    (Sighs with relief)

### Discussion

This initial meeting with Dave was an unsuccessful intake interview. Dave is motivated for therapy, based on his belief that he can mollify his wife's anger over his affair. Unfortunately, his stratagem is only an attempt to manipulate Marie into forgiving him, without his having to take responsibility for his actions. He has no apparent motivation to change his adulterous behavior. In short, there is no basis on which to build a treatment plan.

To recap Jane's three initial interview questions:

1. *Why did this person come here?* In part, he was counting on the confidentiality he expected to keep his secret. In part, he

expected to use the therapist to protect him from further revelations. Meanwhile the fact of being in therapy would give him credible cover with his wife, Marie.

2. *Why did this person come now?* The precipitating event is clear in this case: Dave's deception suddenly revealed by Peggy's call to Marie.

3. *What does this person want?* Dave wanted to "have his cake and eat it too," to hide behind the therapy curtain while continuing to find other partners for brief sexual encounters.

Dave's transparent chicanery provides clear answers to these three questions, but it often takes further exploratory analysis to find the answers.

Jane found it relatively easy to recognize Dave's sociopathy since he seemed unaware of how his statements would sound to her. Identifying sociopathic traits is more difficult when the client is more sophisticated and presents with a carefully curated public persona. This façade of caring about other people, of having a conscience, can persist through the intake process and only become manifest (if it ever does) later in treatment, when it is obvious that the therapy is making little progress and the client has another, hidden agenda.

Jane based her decision not to offer Dave further sessions on four adverse indications. (1) Her recognition of his sociopathic traits leads her to conclude that he would be unable to form a therapeutic alliance: Dave uses relationships with other people to achieve his own ends and lacks the empathic connection with others that would underlie any meaningful connection. (2) He tries to paint himself in a favorable light, but Jane suspects he may be concealing other, more dangerous facts. Jane suspects that Dave's mendacity is part of his standard modus operandum. (3) He would not accept a therapeutic contract based on beneficial changes in his behavior. A false contract—one in which he pretends to accept the need for change but instead uses therapy as a way to placate his wife—would lead either to a treatment impasse or to interminable treatment with no result. (4) Jane's personal dislike for him would impair her ability to be an effective therapist. A therapist tries to offer what Carl Rogers popularized as "unconditional positive regard" as a foundation for the therapeutic alliance (Rogers, 1956). Without this foundation, therapy struggles to succeed.

Jane wondered if her feelings about him represented a counter-transference reaction, based on her own sensitivity to how Dave's "dates" were treated. She decided that it didn't matter: if he elicited that much antipathy in their first meeting, then she was not the therapist for him. Would a male therapist be more understanding of his adultery? Possibly, although it seems unlikely that, given Dave's sociopathic personality, he would benefit from a different therapist or from any psychotherapy.

## Notes

1  See the chapter "General Principles of Psychotherapy."
2  This standard opening question asks, in effect, "What do you want?" and it is important because it establishes that the therapist is offering a service and invites the client
   to begin the negotiation of the treatment contract.
3  Taking notes in front of a client provokes two adverse consequences. (1) It creates
   emotional distance that undermines the therapeutic alliance. (2) It will often distort
   the narrative of clients who modify what they say to conform to the therapist's interests, as revealed by seeing which words the therapist writes down.
4  In the US, the law varies among the states, from an absolute duty to an option to
   warn to merely shielding the practitioner from liability if a warning is given.
5  Matthew 26:41, King James Version, New Testament

## References

Narrow, W. E., Regier, D. A., Rae, D. S., et al. (1993). Use of services of persons with
    mental and addictive disorders: Findings from the National Institute of Mental Health
    Epidemiologic Catchment Area Program. *Archives of General Psychiatry*, 50(2),
    95–107.
Regier, D. A., Narrow, W. E., Rae, D. S., et al. (1993). The de facto US mental and
    addictive disorders service system: Epidemiologic Catchment Area prospective
    1-year prevalence rate of disorders and services. *Archives of General Psychiatry*,
    50(2), 85–94.
Rogers, C. R. (1956). *Client-centered therapy* (3rd ed.). Houghton-Mifflin.

# Dorothy

## A Struggling New Mother

### Referral

Dorothy is self-referred, having heard of Jane from a friend and former patient. Her chief complaint is "since the baby came, I'm having problems with my marriage." She hopes therapy will "show me a way out of all this."

### History

Dorothy gave birth to her first child six months ago at age 33. She has been married for six years. She took medical leave from her job as a court stenographer when she entered her ninth month of pregnancy. Her job provides 12 weeks of paid family medical leave (FML) for the birth and care of a newborn, but she did not return to work after the FML expired. The family is therefore living on her husband's salary as a police officer, a sharp reduction in income. She experienced a few weeks of "the baby blues" after the birth of her son, characterized by weepiness, poor appetite and lack of energy, aggravated by the loss of sleep from four-hour breast feedings and the baby's mild colic.

Dorothy and her husband, Tony, met at the courthouse when he testified in a complicated burglary and assault case in her courtroom. They dated for a year before they married. Tony was promoted to detective five years ago, with an increase in salary but less regular hours. He often works overtime when his case requires it, and now that they have the baby—named Anthony after his father—Tony has been busier than ever and therefore

DOI: 10.4324/9781003353003-11

home even less. Dorothy wonders if he is staying away because Anthony has disrupted their lives and needs so much of her time and attention. She feels Tony has less interest in sex now and that her body has been altered for the worse, first by the pregnancy and now with her breast feeding.

## Mental Status Examination

In her initial interview, Dorothy wore a housedress and sandals. Her hair was messy and her makeup was slapdash. Her overall appearance suggested someone who was not caring for herself. Her speech was soft and whiney and she was tearful in discussing her situation. She had clearly bonded with her baby but also expressed some resentment at the changes his arrival had created in her routines and her marriage, even though she recognized that "I shouldn't blame him. It's not his fault." She denied suicidal ideation and thoughts of harming her child.

## Formulation

The ordinary stresses from the birth of a first child seem to have overwhelmed this otherwise capable and successful woman. At this point it is unclear what vulnerabilities have predisposed her to this reaction but under stress she has regressed to a somewhat helpless state that in turn aggravates her problems. Until further data determine otherwise, her problems appear to be an adjustment reaction that should have a favorable prognosis. Her motivation for therapy and motivation for change are both high.

(Formulation Category: Situational)

## Treatment Plan

The *aim* of therapy will be to help Dorothy regain her prior level of competence, as manifested by her confidence to take care of her baby and to deal with the stresses the marriage has suffered as a result of the new addition to the family. The two *goals* that follow are to bolster her ability to manage the care of her new son and to improve her marital relationship. The *strategy* Jane selects is a cognitive-behavioral approach that may help her to correct the unrealistic self-assessment that she has developed under stress and to view her current situation with more confidence in her abilities. Whether and how much therapeutic attention her marriage may need remains to be assessed. Dorothy readily agrees these are the two areas she is interested in improving. Her agreement completes the *therapeutic contract*. Dorothy agrees to come for weekly sessions to work on these problems.

## SESSION TWO

Dorothy arrives on time and is dressed in a conservative suit. Her hair and makeup are carefully done and she looks much more "put together" than in her first visit. She takes her seat and places her handbag on the floor next to her chair.

Time remaining
45 minutes

Jane          You're looking better today.

*The placebo effect seems already to have helped. Apparently, just talking with Jane at her first meeting has raised her hopes. Jane wants to recognize this change, first, to see if Dorothy agrees and, second, to enhance the improvement by her acknowledgement.*

Dorothy       (Smiles) I feel better. I even thought about canceling for today, but then I decided I better keep the appointment.

Jane          How come?

*She avoids a "why" question.*

Dorothy       Things are better... but not all better. Tony and I are still not the same as before. I'd like to figure out how I got so turned around. I mean, having a baby is a pretty common experience. Why did it throw me for a loop?

Jane    That's a good question. Do you have any beginning answers? Any ideas about what you went through?

> *Dorothy wants to figure out the answer to her question but then asks Jane, the "expert," for it. Jane invites Dorothy to participate in finding solutions to her problems to emphasize the collaborative nature of the therapy and to forestall her thinking that she can passively wait for Jane to supply them.*

Dorothy    (Throws up her hands) I've **been** thinking about it, but I didn't get too far. I mean, I didn't expect a new baby to be so hard. Like I said, millions of women do it every year, yet I couldn't cope. And I thought it would bring Tony and me closer together and instead we're farther apart. (She runs a knuckle under her nose)[1]

Jane    Are you saying there's been **no** improvement with Tony?

> *She challenges Dorothy's all-or-nothing statement as a possible NEGATIVE OVERGENERALIZATION.*

Dorothy    No... Well, a little bit. He's got a lot of unused personal time and comp time from when he was working a case last year where he had to put in a lot of extra hours. So, this week he's been at home more and he helps out with the baby and so that's taken some of the pressure off me.

Jane    Pressure?

*In response to even a subtle challenge, Dorothy responds with a more nuanced and balanced answer. Of the two problem areas—caring for the baby and improving her marital relationship—the former seems more immediate at this point, more important to Dorothy, so Jane elects to focus on that by picking up on the word, "pressure."*

Dorothy  (Raised eyebrows) Well, yeah. My first baby. I don't know what I'm doing. I could screw it up, maybe cause him some permanent problems.

Jane  Permanent problems? Like what?

*Vague worries like "permanent problems" are often impossible to deal with, so Jane asks for specifics. Zeroing in on details is an important TACTIC, not only with cognitive-behavioral therapy but for most therapeutic modalities.*

Dorothy  (Frowns) Like… well, like maybe he'll be screwed up psychologically. Or he won't put on weight the way he's supposed to. When he was colicky, nothing I did would make him feel better. **He** wasn't sleeping. **I** wasn't sleeping. I could have done something wrong and maybe hurt him. (A microexpression appears) I didn't have anyone to tell me how to do it. My family's too far away. My friends are all working… (She trails off, looking helpless)

Jane  You're saying you felt you had to do everything right and you didn't know what the right thing was.

*Jane flags another NEGATIVE OVERGENERALIZATION. Dorothy obviously knows at least some things about caring for Anthony, but she implies that she's totally clueless. Jane thinks the microexpression at the mention of hurting her baby might have been a guilty grimace but she cannot be sure.*

Dorothy   (Winces) No, I didn't. I didn't know anything.

Jane      So one idea that made things hard for you was the belief that you had to do everything right. Be the perfect mother or Anthony would suffer for it.

*By stating the idea so bluntly and using the word "perfect," Jane begins to define the worry as an OVERGENERALIZATION.*

Dorothy   Well, when you say it that way it sounds kind of unrealistic. I know nobody's perfect. I just wanted to do what's best for him.

Jane      Big difference between doing your best and doing everything perfectly.

*Dorothy sounds a little defensive here. Challenging an overgeneralized idea often arouses initial RESISTANCE.*

*Since Dorothy has already picked up the implication, Jane wants to underline it clearly.*

Dorothy   (In a somewhat grudging tone) Yeah…

Jane      Has Anthony been going for checkups with his pediatrician?

*This question and the next lay a FOUNDATION for another approach to the "perfection" issue.*

Dorothy   (Slightly annoyed) Of course.

Jane          How does the doctor think he's doing?

Dorothy       (Reluctantly) She says everything's good. He's grow-
              ing just right on that chart they have.

Jane          When you hear that kind of good report does it
              relieve some of the pressure you've been putting on
              yourself?

              *In other words, have you been a good enough*
              *mother, even if not a perfect one? Another*
              *way of confronting the "perfection" idea.*
              *She repeats Dorothy's term, "pressure,"*
              *matching her* DICTION, *but puts it in the*
              *context of "putting pressure on yourself." Her*
              *restatement with this subtle change includes*
              *the idea that the pressure Dorothy feels is self-*
              *generated rather than created by some ideal of*
              *the perfect mother. She implies that, if Dorothy*
              *is the source of the pressure, then she is the one*
              *who can relieve it.*

Dorothy       You'd think it would, but at first I shrugged it off.
              You know, I read that those doctors spend half their
              time reassuring nervous mothers that everything's all
              right, so I used to tell myself she was just giving me
              the usual line.

              Time remaining
              35 minutes

Jane          And how do **you** think he's doing?

              *Dorothy resists giving up her expectation*
              *of falling short of being the perfect mother,*
              *as if the pediatrician would lie to her. Jane*
              *could challenge this unjustified belief, but*
              *decides it isn't necessary.*

Dorothy    (Shrugs) He's obviously doing fine, so I guess I believe it.

Jane       You guess?

*"Guess" implies that Dorothy has doubts when the evidence is clear that Anthony is thriving. Jane picks up on it to cement the conclusion Dorothy is on the verge of reaching.*

Dorothy    (Grudgingly) Okay. I believe it now.

Jane       So, let's see if we can make sense of this. Your distress was based on what's called an overvalued idea—

*Jane wants to provide Dorothy with the intellectual framework to understand her distorted idea of her performance as a mother. By offering this look at CBT theory, she supports one of the requirements for effective therapy; namely, the patient's "COGNITIVE MASTERY" of the problem.[2]*

Dorothy    A what?

Jane       An overvalued idea. It means an idea that you exaggerate in your mind until it becomes more important than it should be and takes over your thinking. In this case, it was the idea that you had to be the perfect mother or your baby was doomed—

*Jane summarizes it for Dorothy while introducing a NAME for her behavior. NAMING a problem helps a patient understand it better, distance herself from it and see it as manageable. She exaggerates it for stronger effect ("your baby was doomed").*

| | |
|---|---|
| Dorothy | (Laughs and interjects) Well, maybe not "doomed." |
| Jane | —Anything that indicated a problem, like Anthony's colic or his sleep patterns, confirmed it, and the harder you tried to be perfect, the less you thought you succeeded. On top of that, nobody was available to help you figure things out. Not Tony, not your friends, not your mother or anybody in the family. You were all alone facing a complicated challenge and beating yourself up over your supposed failure. |

*She provides Dorothy with an explanation—that she faced it alone, without help from others—that takes the burden off her by suggesting it resulted from circumstances she could not control. This intervention is designed to replace an OVERVALUED IDEA with a more realistic one. Jane also notes that Dorothy has now interrupted her twice, perhaps an indication that she considers herself an equal of Jane, enhancing their desired collaboration.*

| | |
|---|---|
| Dorothy | I could still use a little help. Tony isn't around during the day and at night he can't do much since I'm breast-feeding. It's me that has to get up. |
| Jane | Has your family been any help? |

*Dorothy accepts the explanation, or, at least, doesn't challenge it, and signals this change by agreeing that she hasn't had enough help. Jane follows up with a suggestion in the form of a question. A better question might be, "What other sources of help have you thought about?"*

Dorothy    Well. There's just my mother. I call her sometimes, but she's busy. My brother's no help. (She is flexing her right ankle)[3]

Jane    So you don't see them much?

*Jane has noticed the ankle flexion and takes it as an indication there is something worth exploring about Dorothy's relationship with her mother.*

Dorothy    They visited after Anthony was born. I still send them pictures. But they're too far away to be really helpful.

Jane    So it sounds like there's no real support from the family.

*Jane uses a simple restatement to indicate that she accepts the reality of Dorothy's conclusion.*

Dorothy    (Shakes her head) No, that's right.

Jane    So, let's talk a little more about your mother. It sounds like she's not too available for you.

*She asks specifically about Dorothy's mother to see if it's enough of a problem to warrant more therapy time.*

Dorothy    My mother's not too happy with me. She didn't want me to marry Tony in the first place and I'm not sure she likes the idea that now we have a child.

Jane    What's her problem with Tony?

*Again, she asks for specifics.*

Dorothy    (Shrugs) He didn't go to college. He's a cop. She thinks he's not good enough for me.

Jane       She's said that?

           *She wants to distinguish between what Dorothy thinks is her mother's judgment and what she actually said about Tony.*

Dorothy    Not now, but when I got engaged she was all, "Oh, do you think he's right for you? What if he gets killed?" Stuff like that.

                                                       Time remaining
                                                       25 minutes

Jane       And what did you tell her when she said those things?

           *Jane indicates her interest by asking a further question. She wants to assess whether Dorothy was able to make an independent decision, one that went against her mother's influence.*

Dorothy    I said, yeah, he could be killed but so could anybody. I mean, I'm a court reporter. I see all kinds of trials where bad things happen to people just because they're in the wrong place or they're victims of some crime. At least Tony has a gun and a bunch of other cops looking out for him.

Jane       Was she convinced, your mother? It sounds like you made a pretty strong argument.

           *Jane wants to support Dorothy's successful move toward independence from her family.*

Dorothy    (Raised eyebrows) I don't know if she was convinced, but she shut up about it.

| | |
|---|---|
| Jane | So, then, your mother's not the one you can go to with problems? Is that how you feel? |

*She chooses to focus on the current problem— lack of family support—rather than an old one, family approval of her marriage.*

| | |
|---|---|
| Dorothy | I don't want to give her any more ammunition. And, since my father passed away, she hasn't been the same either. |

| | |
|---|---|
| Jane | How long's he been gone? |

*A piece of information missed in the initial evaluation. Jane wonders how this significant and disruptive event might have figured into the mother–daughter DYNAMIC.*

| | |
|---|---|
| Dorothy | (Her expression saddens) It's six years now. |

| | |
|---|---|
| Jane | So, right around the time you got married? Was it sudden? Had he been ill? |

*Jane makes another connection. She wonders: did her father's death influence her marriage plans or her mother's response? Why didn't Dorothy mention this before?*

| | |
|---|---|
| Dorothy | (Shakes her head) Yeah, he died two months before the wedding. He wasn't sick. They said it was a heart attack. He died in his sleep. We were all really upset about it. Tony thought we might have to postpone the wedding, but I said let's go ahead. |

| | |
|---|---|
| Jane | Do you think that had something to do with how your mother felt about Tony? |

*She presents a possible INTERPRETATION in the form of a question.*

| | |
|---|---|
| Dorothy | I never thought of that. Maybe. |
| Jane | You haven't mentioned your father before. What was he like? Were you close? |

> *Jane decides to ask for additional history to see how her father's death might impact her present problems.*

| | |
|---|---|
| Dorothy | He was an attorney. He did a lot of those cases like you see in the TV ads. Slip and fall, car accidents, that kind of stuff. And no, we weren't close. My brother went to law school. He was the golden child. He was in the practice with my father. Now it's his. |
| Jane | So, your father was distant? Had no time for you? |

> *Jane wonders if her father played any role in the DYNAMICS of her decision to marry Tony.*

| | |
|---|---|
| Dorothy | He was a workaholic. Always in the office or in court. (Bitterly) Unfortunately, he was also an alcoholic, a functioning alcoholic. A lot of these trial lawyers are. It's like a requirement for the job. (Looks up at Jane) You know what? I don't want to talk about them anymore. I've got my own family now. |
| Jane | I can see why you haven't wanted to rely on your mother. |

> *Jane again notices (but does not challenge) how Dorothy feels comfortable changing the subject, another indication of the strength of their collaboration. She abandons the possible new topic to continue to focus on the current difficulty.*

| | |
|---|---|
| Dorothy | Okay. But meanwhile, I've got nobody I can count on. |

Jane            Uh-huh.

                *Jane acknowledges the problem.*

Dorothy        I'm on my own. (She tears up)

Jane            In the past, when it was common for extended families
                to live together, or at least they were close nearby, a
                new mother had her own mother and maybe a grand-
                mother or an aunt or a sister around to help out and
                give advice and share the burdens and the worries.
                Nowadays, that's an unusual arrangement and a lot
                of families are small and on their own, like yours.

                        *Jane makes a NORMATIVE comment with the
                        implication that Dorothy's isolation is not
                        the exception but a common problem. This
                        explanation is an educational statement
                        but it also lays the FOUNDATION for Jane to
                        suggest a possible resource.*

Dorothy        (Shrugs) Nothing I can do about that.

Jane            Maybe you can. Do you use social media at all?

                        *Dorothy defends herself against a criticism
                        Jane did not level at her, suggesting that she
                        still expects herself to be the best possible
                        mother. Jane might have focused on her
                        statement as another OVERGENERALIZATION,
                        but instead she chooses to respond with
                        additional FOUNDATION.*

Dorothy        I'm on Facebook, but since the baby I'm too busy to
                post stuff on my page.

Jane            That might be a source of help for you. A lot of new
                mothers connect on Facebook and use it for support
                and advice.

*Now she can offer a resource and a way
Dorothy can feel less isolated, and perhaps
get some real help, the kind an extended
family might have provided in the past. This
suggestion is an example of briefly utilizing a
CLINICAL CASE MANAGEMENT strategy.*

Dorothy    I've always been leery about putting too much out there on Facebook. When I was working, I had a few trials where somebody got in trouble for stuff they shared or maybe had somebody attack them for it.

Jane    That's true. You do have to be careful. And you might even get some bad advice from other mothers. The question is whether the good outweighs the bad. It's up to you.

*Dorothy's initial RESISTANCE to the suggestion
takes the form of a truthful generalization
that at the same time is actually irrelevant
("Reality is the best resistance" is an old
therapy truism). Jane isn't asking her to post
naked selfies while drunk at a party. Jane
acknowledges Dorothy's concern about social
media, but she tries to make clear that she is
recommending a possible resource, not giving
Dorothy advice either about "mothering" or
even whether to use Facebook for this purpose.*

Dorothy    I'll think about it.

Time remaining
15 minutes

Jane    Okay. Now, what about Tony? You said things are going a little better?

*Dorothy has not committed to using this
resource. Jane's "okay" signals that she's*

*leaving the decision about a Facebook mothers' group up to Dorothy. She switches to a new topic. Jane picks up on Dorothy's initial assertion that she felt better enough after the previous session to consider canceling today's appointment.*

Dorothy    (Nods) They are a little better, actually.

Jane    How so?

*Dorothy accepts the change of topic. Jane needs details and facts to work with, but she avoids a "why" question with another phrase.*

Dorothy    Like I said, he's been home more and helping out, but we're not back to how things were before.

Jane    "Before" when?

*Jane assumes Dorothy means before the pregnancy, but she wants to be sure about this important issue.*

Dorothy    Before the baby. Or, actually, before I got pregnant.

Jane    Can you tell me more about that?

*In order to offer any meaningful intervention, Jane knows she will need a clear idea about their relationship.*

Dorothy    Sooo… We were married for four, almost five, years before I got pregnant, and things were good. Maybe not as lovey-dovey as when we first started out, but he was still interested in sex. We had fun. We went out. We saw friends. Both of us were working so we had more money.

Jane        And now?

*Another brief phrase to show her continuing interest and to encourage further details.*

Dorothy     Now we don't do any of that.

Jane        No sex?

*She asks about the most significant element of Dorothy's list.*

Dorothy     Not since I was six months pregnant.

Jane        So that's what? Nine months!

*Her emphasis is designed to elicit more information.*

Dorothy     Feels like even longer. I mean, at first, I wasn't interested. Not when I was big as a horse and then when I was just starting to learn what I had to do for Anthony. I was so exhausted, sex was the last thing on my mind. But now I miss it and he seems like he lost interest.

Jane        And what about the rest of the relationship, other than the sex part?

*She wants to fill in the other list of changes since Anthony's birth to get a more complete picture before focusing on the change in their sexual relationship.*

Dorothy     (Looks hurt) Not as good either. He's friendly, but distant.

| Jane | Any ideas about why? |
|------|------|

*She asks Dorothy to collaborate on the problem.*

| Dorothy | I don't know. Maybe he doesn't want the baby now. Maybe it's something with his work. I just don't know. |
|------|------|

| Jane | Wouldn't he want the baby? His namesake. |
|------|------|

*The idea that Tony rejects the baby, although stated casually, suggests a deep worry about a CATASTROPHIC DYNAMIC. Jane has to deal with it immediately.*

| Dorothy | (Bitterly) Yeah, right. Anthony, Jr. |
|------|------|

| Jane | Here's something to think about. Before Anthony came along, you and Tony were a pair. Now you're a trio and you have to divide your attention between two people in the family instead of just Tony. That's a big change. How do you think that affects him? |
|------|------|

*Jane could pick up on a possible conflict about naming their baby or even the tone of contempt she reveals toward Tony about his desire to have a namesake. Instead, she keeps to the topic and provides an alternate, more benign explanation.*

| Dorothy | He's never said anything about that. You think he's feeling neglected? |
|------|------|

| Jane | It might be hard for him to acknowledge he resents his own son, even to himself. |
|------|------|

*Dorothy picks up on Jane's question in a way that suggests she may have understood*

*Tony's feelings without consciously recognizing them. Jane takes a chance in suggesting what Tony might be feeling, since she's never met him and her only "version" of Tony is the one provided by Dorothy.*

Dorothy    Maybe that's it. What should I do about it?

Jane    What do you think you **could** do?

*Even with the "maybe" it's likely that this idea has resonated with Dorothy. Her request for advice confirms it. Jane declines to provide any idea about what she should do, rejecting Dorothy's request for answers, but using a question that invites her to collaborate in figuring out a possible solution.*

Dorothy    (Annoyed) And why should it be up to me? It's his problem.

Jane    Maybe it is, but Tony isn't here. It's just you and me. So, the only way we can try to change things with him, and between the two of you, is if you change toward him. Think of it as two people dancing the two-step—

*Dorothy rejects the invitation. If she can't get an answer from Jane she wants Tony to take responsibility. Jane wants to emphasize her point so she begins to use a metaphor, a form of RHETORIC.*

Dorothy    (Grimaces) The two-step? What's that?

Jane    A kind of slow dancing. The partners are holding each other and sliding one foot and then bringing the other foot after it.

*Unfortunately, Dorothy doesn't recognize the metaphor. Because of the unforeseen error in* DICTION, *Jane has to stop and explain her symbolism. That weakens the effect but Jane persists.*

Dorothy     (Laughs) Oh, yeah. I've seen that in a movie. A western, I think it was.

Jane        (Smiles) Ok, I didn't say it was a modern dance step, but bear with me. Think of two people dancing the two-step and then one of them changes to a foxtrot and then again to a waltz. The other dancer has to change each time. So, you and Tony are doing the two-step but if you change, he'll have to change as well.

            *Even though it's a clumsy metaphor, the best she could think of in the moment, Jane hopes it helps get her point across in a way that will stick in Dorothy's mind.*

Dorothy     (Nods) Well, that makes sense.

Jane        Could you start by actually discussing it with him, how you feel about him? Do you have that kind of relationship?

            *Since Dorothy accepts the idea Jane tries to consolidate and extend it.*

Dorothy     Maybe. We're not big on heart-to-heart stuff. You know, Tony's kind of the strong, silent type.

Jane        Hmm. Can you tell me more about Tony?

            *What Dorothy chooses to say about him and her interpretation of his background will differ from what his mother might say or one*

*of his fellow police detectives. Asking for
Dorothy's perception of her husband is, then,
another way of looking into the nature of their
relationship.*

Dorothy    Tony? I don't… well, he's, uh… What do you want
to know?

Jane       Just what kind of guy he is, where'd he grow up, just
whatever you think is important about him.

> *Two of the three criteria will depend on
> Dorothy's perception.*

Dorothy    Okay. Well, he grew up in Nebraska. The family has a
farm there. Two brothers and a sister. He's the second
oldest. Um… he enlisted in the Army after high school.
He went to Fort Leonard Wood for training as military
police and then he was stationed in California. He hurt
his knee. They were playing football on the base and
he tripped and did something to his knee, so he was on
limited duty for a while and then they let him out early
with a disability, ten per cent, but he was really okay so
they took him into the police here… That's about it.

Jane       What about his family in Nebraska? Do you see much
of them?

> *Dorothy chooses to list Tony's historical
> data over a personal description. Jane could
> explore this "distancing" further but they are
> near the end of the session. She elects to gather
> more history. Relationships with in-laws can
> reflect Dorothy's own view of Tony.*

Dorothy    (Speaks in a flat tone) No, not since the wedding. I
mean, we were married here and they all came for

that. We did go out there once for a visit. His mother calls every so often, but other than that, no, we don't.

Jane  And Tony? What's his relationship with the family like?

> *Jane persists on the topic even though Dorothy doesn't seem very interested in it. How Tony reacts to his family could also reveal how she sees him.*

Dorothy  (Impassively) He loves them. But they're just too far away.

Jane  How about Tony's friends? What are they like?

> *Dorothy is sticking with bare facts and historical data, not giving Jane the picture she wants her to paint. Jane recognizes her apparent disinterest, but, not knowing the cause, keeps to the topic. A METACOMMUNICATION is indicated, something that acknowledges Dorothy's mechanical recital, even one as simple as, for instance, "You sound like you're not too interested in this topic." Letting Dorothy drone on when she is so clearly disengaged wastes time without advancing the therapy.*

Dorothy  (Looks at the ceiling) They're all police, too. He plays basketball with a group of them. Sometimes we go out with them. Not since the baby came.

Jane  We talked about how you didn't have any family support. Would you say the same for Tony?

> *She tries to focus in on Tony's reaction to the baby.*

| Dorothy | I never thought about that, but, yeah, I guess that's right. Doesn't seem to bother him though… (She suddenly looks more intense) Look, there's something I need to tell you. Something bad. |

Time remaining
5 minutes

| Jane | Okay. |

*Evidently, this new topic is why she wasn't interested in talking about Tony. Again, an earlier* METACOMMUNICATION *might have brought up the new topic sooner. Now it sounds like Dorothy is about to make a confession. If so, it indicates her trust in Jane and the strength of the* THERAPEUTIC ALLIANCE. *Jane makes a neutral response rather than commenting on the "something bad" statement.*

| Dorothy | (Hangs her head) Back when Anthony was having all that colic trouble, he wouldn't stop crying. Nothing I did ever worked. Rocking him, walking him. Singing to him even. He just cried and cried. (She stops and stares at the wall) So, then, this one time, I just couldn't take it anymore and I… slapped him. |

| Jane | Slapped? |

*Jane asks about the ambiguous word: does slapped mean an open hand blow or something more?*

| Dorothy | Yeah. So, of course, he started crying worse and I picked him up and tried to soothe him and eventually he stopped and fell asleep. |

| Jane | (Remains quiet) |

*When faced with a confession, she wants to let it all come out before responding to it.*

Dorothy    Well, aren't you going to say anything?

Jane    What are you expecting me to say?

*Jane sidesteps the question by asking one in return. Dorothy seems to want Jane to judge her or perhaps absolve her of her guilt, both stances Jane wants to avoid in favor of a collaborative response.*

Dorothy    (Anguished) I don't know. Just say something.

Jane    I can see that you feel very guilty and ashamed about what happened.

*She chooses to acknowledge Dorothy's feelings rather than to judge her behavior.*

Dorothy    I do. It only happened that once. I never told Tony I did it.

Jane    So it's been weighing on you.

*Again, she describes Dorothy's emotional response but says nothing about the act itself. So far, Jane has not assessed whether the baby is at risk from an abusive parent.*

Dorothy    I'm afraid it might happen again.

Jane    Have you had other times when you had the impulse to hit him?

*Now she begins to assess the risk.*

Dorothy    (Shakes her head) No.

Jane        We can talk more about that next time, if you like, but
            our time is up for today and we have to stop.

            *Dorothy's denial is somewhat reassuring
            and if time permitted Jane might have
            pursued it further.*

### Discussion

Patients often wait until near the end of the session to bring up material that is fraught in order to limit the perceived risk. If the therapist extends the session it creates a precedent that may be difficult to reverse. Recognizing that time was short, Jane focused on risk assessment rather than her patient's feelings. She was somewhat reassured by Dorothy's denial of any more instances of hitting her baby, but she will need to revisit the topic.

In this session, Jane was able to address both of Dorothy's problem areas: feeling overwhelmed with a new baby and the marital rift between her and Tony. Her challenge to a negative overgeneralization (I'm useless because I can't take care of my baby) brought out new material. Another overly pessimistic idea (I'm all alone with nobody who can help me) belied her report that Tony was home more and helping with the baby. Dorothy seemed receptive to the reality points Jane provided, a hopeful sign that she is responding well to the therapy.

To counter this self-defeating perception, Jane suggested using social media as a resource; specifically, looking for a mother's group on Facebook. The suggestion required a change of therapeutic strategy, from CBT to clinical case management (Kanter, 1989). Jane knows mothers use Facebook successfully in this way. Instead of advice she suggests a resource. She was able to make this suggestion because Dorothy is a relatively mature and competent person who seems unlikely to develop an overdependency on Jane, even though Jane acted here as if she was Dorothy's missing mother.

The second half of the session then focused on Dorothy's dissatisfaction with her marital relationship. She was able to counter

Dorothy's cognitive error (Tony is no longer interested in me) with a more hopeful alternative (Tony feels abandoned by your preoccupation with the new baby) that suggested a possible solution (correct Tony's idea by showing how you feel about him). By placing the responsibility on Dorothy, Jane hopes this idea may give her a sense of control over her marital problem. It makes Dorothy the active change agent instead of the passive victim of circumstances. Whether she can adopt either of these strategies and whether they will be helpful remains to be seen.

An important development in this session was the recognition that Dorothy and Tony have made a successful transition from their parental families (the families of origin) to a self-contained, stable unit (the family of procreation). This independent status suggests they will be able to transcend their current stresses and continue to build a stable relationship.

## SESSION THREE

One week later. Dorothy enters the office briskly. Her posture and bearing look more confident than on the two previous occasions. She is again dressed in a business suit with low heels. She heads straight for her chair and sits alertly into her seat. This body-language behavior suggests to Jane that she is feeling more in control and better about herself.

Time remaining
45 minutes

Jane      So, let's see. Why don't we pick up with where we left off? You were telling me about that time you slapped Anthony.

*Although she was reassured by Dorothy's contention at the end of the previous session, she needs to complete her assessment of the potential for harm to the baby.*

| Dorothy | You know, I felt better after I told you about that. Even though it was just that one time. I couldn't believe I did that. That's just not me. |

| Jane | So it never happened again? |
| | *Evidently, her confession has helped Dorothy accept what happened without continuing to castigate herself for it. Jane double-checks on what Dorothy said last week.* |

| Dorothy | It didn't. (Grimaces) I was just so frazzled back then, I didn't know what I was doing. I must have been crazy from lack of sleep and all the stress I was under. I would never hurt my baby. |

| Jane | I'm glad to hear that. |
| | *Awarding her approval (or disapproval) to something a patient has done can be problematic. It can increase dependence, stir up TRANSFERENCE issues or provoke RESISTANCE. Given the importance of this issue, Jane chooses to reinforce her behavior.* |

| Dorothy | Yeah. I never told Tony about that night. He would have gone ballistic. |

| Jane | How are things with Tony? |
| | *Reassured, for now, about the risk of child abuse, Jane moves on.* |

| Dorothy | (Smiles) Better, actually. I tried to do what you said and it seemed to help. |

| Jane | (Nods) So it seems promising? |

*First, Jane didn't "say" she should talk*
*to Tony. She **asked** if she felt comfortable*
*doing so. Telling her to do it might have*
*created* RESISTANCE. *Second, "seemed"*
*implies that she is not ready to claim victory*
*or commit herself to a judgment. Dorothy's*
*body language and voice tone, however, both*
*suggest she is more confident than her actual*
*words would suggest. Jane wants to keep her*
*on topic. She acknowledges the ambivalence*
*and reinforces the idea of progress.*

Dorothy    (Shrugs) I was pretty nervous at first. Tony had a couple of days off, so we had breakfast together. Hadn't done that in a long time. And I said to him that I thought he'd been unhappy lately and he said work's been busy and I said what about here at home.

Jane    So you didn't let him divert away from your point.

*Again, she supports Dorothy by recognizing*
*her attempt to keep the discussion going where*
*she needs it to. The more effective response*
*might have been to say nothing: Dorothy*
*didn't seem uncertain or hesitant and so*
*perhaps she didn't need the extra prodding or*
*reinforcement. A symbolic "pat on the head"*
*may foster dependency on the therapist.*

Dorothy    No. So then I said, it's been hard with a new baby and I've been having a rough time figuring out how to take care of him. Then he got kind of defensive and said he was trying to help all he could. And I said I knew he was and I appreciated it, but it was still hard for me. But then I realized I was talking about me and not about him, so I wasn't sure where to go with it next. (She pauses and looks at the floor. Jane waits and lets the silence build.) So, breakfast was over and he went out to mow the lawn and I went up to take care of Anthony.

Jane      And then?

*By continuing to express her interest in the narrative Jane both keeps her on topic and maintains her support.*

Dorothy   I thought about it some more and when he came back in from mowing the lawn I said I wanted to talk some more about what I said at breakfast. We went back in the kitchen and I made coffee. So then I told him I had talked to you about things. I mean, after I saw you last week he asked me how did it go and I said okay but I didn't go into any detail and he didn't ask so I thought I better say more about it.

Jane      What did you tell him?

*Bringing up her professional, Jane, suggests Dorothy lacks the confidence to carry on the discussion on her own. Evidently, she felt she needed Jane to back her up. Jane wants to know to what extent Dorothy needed to use Jane's "expert" status to deal with Tony.*

Dorothy   I said you suggested that he was having trouble adjusting to the new baby too and that I hadn't thought about that before but it made sense that Anthony would make a difference in our relationship. And he said were you blaming him? And he looked annoyed. So I said not at all. You were saying that we had to adjust from being just a couple to being a family and that both of us had to make the adjustment, not only me. He thought about that, sort of staring at the table and then he said he thought that was right and what did you say we should do about it.

Jane       Sounds like I was the silent partner in this discussion.

*With this* METACOMMUNICATION, *she acknowledges Dorothy's use of her authority without criticizing her for it.*

Dorothy     (Shrugs) I couldn't think how else to bring it up.

Time remaining
35 minutes

Jane       What happened next?

*Dorothy's defensive statement shows she is aware that she needed help. Again, Jane uses a neutral question to show Dorothy she is not judging her. What she wants to convey is the idea that Dorothy doesn't need her expert backing, but her response doesn't yet accomplish that.*

Dorothy     We talked some more and then he went up to take a shower 'cause he was sweaty after mowing and I went up too and we ended up in bed. (Grins) So that was at least one good thing that came out of it.

Jane       The whole thing sounds like it went pretty well.

*"It went" reinforces her in her success, without saying "you" did pretty well, which might have come across as condescending.*

Dorothy     Yeah, it did.

| Jane | And how's it going with the other man in your life? |
| --- | --- |

*Still controlling the agenda, Jane asks about the other treatment GOAL, her feeling overwhelmed with caring for her first baby.*

| Dorothy | With Anthony? That's going better. I took your advice and went on Facebook. It's amazing how much is there for women with new babies. With babies in general. I got into a group of maybe a dozen new mothers, women with young kids. I guess I should have known this but we're all having the same problems. I got some good ideas, too. |
| --- | --- |

| Jane | Sounds like it's been a good week all around. |
| --- | --- |

*Jane didn't directly give her "advice" about Facebook; rather, she made her aware of a possible resource. At this point, however, nothing useful would come from her pointing out the subtle difference, so she lets it go.*

| Dorothy | (Nods) It has. |
| --- | --- |

| Jane | All right, let's take stock of where we are. We had two areas where you were having difficulty, right? You were feeling overwhelmed with the new baby and there was tension between you and Tony. |
| --- | --- |

*Jane somewhat downplays the intensity of the problems in the way she characterizes them. Her intention here is to see if Dorothy still needs her help.*

| Dorothy | I don't know about "tension." I thought we were headed for divorce. |
| --- | --- |

Jane        Really? I don't recall that you used that word.

*Dorothy recognizes that Jane is understating her problems and responds by overstating it. Jane challenges her on it.*

Dorothy     Maybe I didn't use it, but I sure thought it.

Jane        What do you think now?

*She wants to assess how much has changed for the better and whether they have met the therapy GOALS.*

Dorothy     Now? I don't think we're headed that way.

Jane        So, you and Tony, you're on a good path?

*She tries to confirm the progress.*

Dorothy     Yeah, we are.

Jane        Things are better?

*Jane is at a decision point. The TREATMENT CONTRACT on which they agreed had two GOALS and it appears both have been met. That success should result in the termination of therapy. Jane knows from experience, however, that patients, especially when therapy has been helpful, may be reluctant for it to end. She wants to be sure before making a decision about further therapy.*

Dorothy     (Nods) Things are definitely better with us.

Jane

Okay, so the two areas we decided to work on are both going better. What would you think of us waiting to see how things go before making another appointment?

> *Jane hopes Dorothy can continue her progress on her own, which would both strengthen her self-confidence and head off her becoming dependent on Jane, perhaps in a surrogate "grandmother" role.*

Dorothy

(Looks horrified) What! You're throwing me out?

Jane

(Holds up both hands, palms out) No, just the opposite. I'm saying, you're doing so well, maybe you don't need more therapy at this point. You need time to consolidate the gains you've made.

> *The abrupt suggestion has startled Dorothy, who may already have been expecting Jane to continue to be her expert backup. Because of Dorothy's turmoil and anxiety, Jane tries to emphasize the positive side of her suggestion.*

Dorothy

(Anxiously) But what if I don't? What if things don't go well?

Jane

You can always come back. In fact, you don't have to be floundering to see me again. If you just want to review what's happening or bring me up to date you could make an appointment and come in.

> *Dorothy begins to REGRESS to the helpless state in which she began treatment, even though she has obviously overcome her earlier feelings of being weak and vulnerable. Jane tries to assert the reality of her suggestion: she is not*

*abandoning Dorothy. She has made significant
progress but is able to return whenever she
needs or wants to.*

Dorothy    (Shaking her head) I don't know. I mean, I'm not
even back to work yet. I used up my family leave
days and now I'm on unpaid vacation. We're living
on one paycheck. With Anthony in the picture our
budget's increased. Tony's taking all the overtime he
can get and that helps but it's not making up for my
salary. What am I going to do about all that?

Jane    That's a problem we didn't talk about at the beginning, isn't it?

*Jane acknowledges that Dorothy still has
"unfinished business," even if it was not
part of the original* THERAPEUTIC CONTRACT.
*Although Dorothy does not think about it
that way, what she has raised is a question of
whether the contract can be "renegotiated"
into a new agreement with the* GOAL *of her
return to work.*

Dorothy    We didn't, not specifically, but that's always been a
question. Maybe there was too much else to worry
about then and we didn't consider it but it's still a
problem.

Time remaining
25 minutes

Jane    That's true. So, what is your plan about going back
on the job?

*Jane is willing to see if they need to work
on this new issue, but she wants to know*

*what Dorothy's thinking is first. Is it really a problem? If so, how big?*

| | |
|---|---|
| Dorothy | I… I don't have a plan. Just a lot of questions. Should I go back at all? I have seniority and it pays well. I have a lot of job security there. So that's one thing. But if I go back now, who's going to take care of Anthony? He's too young for daycare. He's only seven months. I can't bring him to work. I'm usually in court all day. I can't ask the judge to call a recess just so I can go take care of my baby. So there's that. And I'm still breast-feeding. That's another question. What do I do about that? I read where some mothers use a breast pump to switch to bottles. But who's going to give him the bottle? Arggh. (She buries her face in her hands) |
| Jane | It is a lot of questions. How much have you been thinking about them at this point? |

*Jane recognizes the reality of her concerns but also wants to acknowledge that it may be too early to try to answer them. She thinks Dorothy is focused on them now because of the possible therapy termination. It's like she's saying, "Don't abandon me now because I still need lots of help."*

| | |
|---|---|
| Dorothy | I didn't think I had to. I thought we'd have time to deal with them later. |
| Jane | It sounds like you feel you couldn't solve these issues on your own. |

*This METACOMMUNICATION is designed to confront Dorothy with the question of why she needs Jane. On the one hand, her*

> *anxiety about proceeding on her own shows how strong the THERAPEUTIC ALLIANCE now is. On the other hand, it suggests that she may be developing an unhealthy dependency on Jane. It is an important distinction for Jane to know if she should continue the therapy with this new GOAL or try to reassure Dorothy that she can function without her.*

Dorothy    I don't know if I can.

Jane    My thought that we could finish up is based on how well you've done with the problems we started with, and in a relatively short time, too. But it seems like my confidence in you is greater than your confidence in yourself.

> *Jane states the problem overtly to see which side Dorothy will come down on. Either she has confidence in her own abilities or she doesn't.*

Dorothy    I don't know. I don't know how I feel about that.

Jane    When do you think the question will have to be answered? Or, let me put it another way: when will you need the money from your job badly enough that you'll be forced to make a decision?

> *Jane tries a new tack to see how relevant the job question is at the present moment.*

Dorothy    We're getting by at the moment but it's tight. And we have some savings that we might have to use, although I'd hope not.

| | |
|---|---|
| Jane | So, let me see if I understand what you're saying. The job question is a tough one, but you have too many advantages to give up your position at the court. Anthony might still be too young to change his care now. You're getting by on one paycheck but it's a strain. You don't know how long you can go without your salary. Have I covered everything? |

*Jane summarizes the discussion to lay a FOUNDATION.*

| | |
|---|---|
| Dorothy | I think so. |

| | |
|---|---|
| Jane | So, all those questions are actually practical issues. By that I mean, they're not psychological. Or not on their face, even though there might be psychological issues underlying them. But they're hard decisions to make. So, I guess what I'm getting at is, how do you think therapy can help you with them? |

*If Jane is to continue therapy with Dorothy she wants a clear idea of what they would try to accomplish. Otherwise, they might slide into a long-term arrangement where Dorothy feels she needs to keep talking to Jane about whatever is going on in her life.*

| | |
|---|---|
| Dorothy | I get what you're saying. I'm just not ready to stop. |

| | |
|---|---|
| Jane | We can continue to meet, but we'll have to decide what it is we're working on. |

*Jane recognizes that they will need additional time to WORK THROUGH the question of further therapy.*

Dorothy        Sounds good.

Jane           Well, how about this: let's meet next week again as
               scheduled and meanwhile you can think about it and
               we'll see how things look then.

               *Termination, even after such a short course
               of treatment, often is a difficult phase of the
               therapy. Jane isn't sure at this point how
               long it will take.*

Dorothy        Okay.

Time remaining
12 minutes

Jane           Good. Well, let's stop for today and I'll see you next
               week.

               *Jane ends the session early and doesn't use
               her usual time-is-up-and-we-have-to-stop
               formula. Stopping a little early reinforces
               her suggestion that Dorothy doesn't need her
               to make further progress.*

### Discussion

This short, concentrated period of treatment shows how a determined patient with emotional intelligence and interpersonal skills
can rather quickly put herself on the road to recovery. The rapid resolution of Dorothy's situational problems demonstrates that a patient
highly motivated to change can utilize therapeutic work to achieve
significant progress. Moreover, therapeutic advances gain momen-
tum that often brings about further improvement in the weeks and
months ahead after the formal sessions have ended. Knowing of this
carry-over effect gives Jane more confidence in her decision to stop.

Dorothy considered canceling the second session because
she was feeling better, only to react strongly to the idea that she
didn't need further therapy when Jane suggested they could stop.

Termination, even after a short period of treatment, can often be difficult. Dorothy may cancel the next appointment and end the therapy herself. She might return with a new set of "problems" in order to prolong therapy.

Even after just three meetings, Dorothy is becoming dependent on Jane. When patients establish they are capable of handling their problem areas without therapy support, there is, nevertheless, the danger of turning a short-term treatment into a long-term, "interminable" supportive relationship in which the patient becomes less self-reliant and unhealthily dependent on the therapist.

Jane maintained a sharp focus on the two therapy goals. Prior to the birth of her son, Dorothy had a successful marital relationship and held a skilled and responsible position as a court stenographer. Under the stress of caring for a new baby, with no prior experience or supportive family to help cushion the stress, she regressed to an anxious, needy and insecure state. She began to improve immediately, perhaps because she viewed Jane as a source of help and support before Jane had offered any, a placebo effect. She made immediate and effective use of the initiatives brought up in the second session and by the third was well on her way to reclaiming her prior level of function. What remained was for Jane to help her let go of the therapy and continue to use her abilities on her own. How many more sessions this might take is unclear, but maybe no more than one or two.

The new treatment contract Dorothy proposed was based on practical and monetary questions that would usually be outside the purview of therapy. Another treatment contract, one with appropriate goals, is a possibility. Perhaps it would deal with any residual problems Dorothy had from her family of origin, her alcoholic and emotionally distant father, for example. A second period of therapy can be justified if problems that were originally obscured by the present crisis become more prominent as those initial problems are resolved. Dorothy did not take this path. She did not want to discuss her family when Jane inquired about them and she did not raise any of those old issues when Jane brought up termination.

Sometimes a long period of therapy can be a series of successful efforts to deal with a hierarchy of problems. This approach only works, however, if it involves genuine areas of difficulty and is not a covert effort by the therapist to keep patients in treatment because of the comfort of an established relationship or the financial incentive of reliable payments.

## Notes

1 The "nose wipe" is a non-verbal signal of disapproval.
2 See the chapter "General Principles of Psychotherapy."
3 A non-verbal indication of tension about this topic.

## Reference

Kanter, J. W. (1989). Clinical case management: Definition, principles, components. *Hospital and Community Psychiatry*, 40(4), 361–368.

# Epilogue

## Review

Jane applied her methodological skills to help eight diverse individuals with a variety of clinical challenges, typical of an established psychotherapy practice.

- Four presented with apparent *developmental* delays, but subsequent information modified three of these initial formulations. George, after revealing his voyeurism, faced *transactional* and *psychodynamic* difficulties. Sophie first presented with a late adulthood *developmental* transition; then revealed a *situational* area of conflict regarding her sexuality. Martin's initial presentation of a *developmental* transition of early adulthood quickly revealed he had significant *transactional* and *psychodynamic* challenges as well. Only Holly continued to face an essentially *developmental* task, although some *transactional* issues began to arise with regard to her interactions with her husband.
- Three initially presented with *situational* difficulties, but, again, with further history, one formulation had to be modified and the other turned out to be a false front. Ellen's work-related troubles shaded into a *psychodynamic* framework. Dave's story was only a cover for his covert non-therapeutic agenda. Only Dorothy successfully overcame the *situational* hardships of her post-partum struggles.
- One client, Charles, appeared to confront an *existential* threat but Jane had overlooked a significant *situational* trauma related to his Covid-19 illness.

DOI: 10.4324/9781003353003-12

- Missing from this group was anyone with a *biological* presentation or with a *dissociative* disorder. In the treatment of biological illness, medication and other non-therapy measures may take precedence, although psychotherapy can be a helpful adjunct. In fact, studies have shown that cognitive-behavioral therapy is as effective as antidepressant medication and may have better long-term benefits (Driessen & Hollon, 2019). Dissociative disorders are either rare, like fugue states or dissociative identity disorder (formerly called "multiple personality"), or they require specific treatment protocols, as with post-traumatic stress disorder, and are not frequently seen in office practice.
- These clinical examples illustrate the usefulness of a formulation in planning a successful therapy. They also demonstrate the importance of modifying a formulation when new clinical data emerge in the course of treatment.

## What Happens Next?

Because each patient record covered only one or two sessions, it is tempting to speculate about the future success or failure of the members of this disparate group. How would they have fared as they continued in treatment? What might happen if they did not? What were the ultimate outcomes of their therapeutic experiences? Predictions about their future can only involve educated guesses.

- *Holly: a promising beginning.* Holly's challenge is to separate from her parent's family while achieving a better balance of power in her new marriage. In this transitional period of her life, Holly is evolving a different identity. It is based on the strong role model provided by her mother, who stayed home to raise the children but then went out into the working world against the wishes of her traditional husband. If she can assert herself without fracturing her relationship with her own traditional husband, Holly could become someone who makes independent life choices. Among them: how close to remain with the family in which she grew up, when and if to have children, and whether to work in the home or outside of it.

- *George: a failed treatment due to the therapist's misjudgment.* George came into therapy with a subsidiary set of problems supposedly arising from uncertainty about his position as a graduate student in the Divinity School. In his fifth session, however, Jane was surprised to learn that he had an encounter with the police because of voyeurism. Without this near-arrest experience, George might never have brought up this important problem and Jane suspected it was not his only prevarication. Unfortunately, after this uncomfortable session, George fled from therapy. With the advantage of hindsight, Jane realized she had overreacted to this disclosure. She assumed that George agreed with the new treatment contract she proposed, an agreement based on his need to control his impulse disorder. She immediately launched into an aggressive behavior modification program with a set of tactics she hoped would allow him to restrain his paraphilic impulses. Even though he appeared to accept the new plan, his subsequent actions made it clear that George could not tolerate the new approach. Chances are almost certain that his voyeurism will continue. It may be that his next encounter with a behavioral health service will be mandated by a court.

- *Ellen: short-term success and long-term uncertainty.* Ellen appeared able to regulate her behavior at work to improve her performance and, incidentally, to avoid being fired. Jane's focus on the underlying personality traits and the way they create unnecessary problems for Ellen will meet resistance from Ellen's difficulty appreciating these ego syntonic habits as problems that need to change. They are not likely to yield to short-term therapy. Jane's challenge will be to remain effectively focused on the personality modifications and to avoid the distractions Ellen will present as she tries to use the sessions to vent and find a sympathetic ear for her frustrations. The tension between the two types of content may only be resolved after many sessions. The risk is that therapy might devolve into a long-term "supportive" process without further benefit.

- *Charles: a flawed formulation delays recognition of the precipitating event.* Jane overlooked Charles' harrowing experience with a Covid-19 infection until well into the second therapy session. Now that Jane has identified his recent illness as the source of Charles's end-of-life ruminations, she will be more focused on the impact of this event and less responsive to general, nonspecific existential issues. Charles' sessions were marked by an unusual intellectualism manifested, for example, by the appearance of literary quotations. Jane mirrored Charles's diction with her own quotes as a way to connect with him more successfully and to strengthen the therapeutic alliance. A partial breakthrough occurred because of the death of the family pet. Charles allowed himself an emotional response and made an important and hopeful step forward with his plan to adopt a new puppy. Charles may need at least several more sessions before he can resume the activities and interests of his retirement.
- *Sophie: a successful brief therapy.* Sophie seemed more in charge of the agenda than Jane, whose main contribution was as an empathetic listener. Jane's non-judgmental attitude and the safe environment of the office were the agencies that facilitated this brief therapy. Sophie seemed quite muddled at the beginning but was able, with the help of a passage from a book she found deeply meaningful, to formulate her own case and work it through to a solution in a short time. She seems firmly on a path to attain her personal and educational goals.
- *Martin: a long-term struggle.* One might expect Martin to be the most promising client: young, intelligent, motivated. On the contrary, Jane can anticipate slow going with this lonely young man who has already had four years of psychoanalysis without any significant benefit. Now every therapy session feels like a struggle. Martin uses his impressive intellectual gifts to resist Jane's therapeutic efforts. Unless Jane can head him off, Martin could become one of those patients for whom being in therapy

is the reason he stays in therapy, a persistent "patient" but with no meaningful change in his behavior. Jane will have to work hard to prevent that outcome and it may require another extended period of treatment.

- *Dave: an untreatable sociopath.* Jane could not offer this man treatment that would, in effect, represent her collusion in his scheme to placate and deceive his wife. Without motivation to change, Dave will likely continue as a serial adulterer. His antisocial personality traits might negatively affect his wife and children and perhaps will get him into trouble at his real estate job; for example, if he helps himself to the firm's escrow account or misrepresents a property in order to make a sale.

- *Dorothy: success in overcoming situational stress.* A short period of high stress related to the birth of her first child overwhelmed the defenses of this capable and accomplished woman. Dorothy was able to take advantage of Jane's insightful assessment and therapeutic interventions to quickly bring her problems under control. Paradoxically, her success created a strong dependency on Jane, but once that is resolved, Dorothy should be fine on her own.

## Themes

Two concepts that run through this book are (1) the question of the proper length of a course of psychotherapy and (2) the therapist's decision-making process about what kind of treatment to offer.

This eight-person sample is notable for the wide variation in the anticipated length of treatment. How long a course of psychotherapy should be remains both a troubling economic and an unsettled theoretical issue. Private insurance, employer plans and government benefits are all interested in the lowest cost of treatment and base their calculations on the length of time or number of services they must cover. Unlike some health care services, however, the time needed for a completed course of psychotherapy is often unpredictable. In the face of this uncertainty, third-party payors have tried to achieve predictability by reducing the amount they will pay for a session, limiting the number of visits they will pay for and instituting prior authorization requirements. The United States Congress has enacted legislation from 1996 through 2022 mandating parity between behavioral health and other health services, such as medical and surgical care, but so far these laws seem to have had little impact (HHS Press Office, 2022). The problem continues to be the ongoing cost of long-term treatment.

Long-term treatment can result from a failure to end the therapy when the goals of the treatment plan have been met. As mentioned earlier, factors such as a reluctance to discharge a familiar patient or to give up the financial benefit of an established "income stream" can negatively impact the therapist's judgment, often to the patient's detriment. In at least two instances, however, long-term therapy is not only justified but actually necessary:

- The first is those clients whose therapy is directed primarily at maladaptive personality traits that tend to be ego syntonic. Change is often slow and requires a long period of working through.
- The second is the treatment of patients whose own defenses and ability to cope with the ordinary stresses of life are inadequate to the task. The therapist provides the support and guidance these people need to function successfully. Technically, the therapist acts as an *auxiliary ego* who furnishes the executive functions the client is unable to acquire or exercise for themselves.

In these two exceptional situations, therapy is prolonged and, if the patient requires an auxiliary ego, may last as long as the therapist is in practice. Perhaps the most practical approach to this vexing question of treatment duration is to see it in parallel with a medical model. Medical illnesses can be acute or chronic and sometimes relapsing illnesses require multiple periods of active treatment. Behavioral health problems that receive professional treatment will also require acute treatment and sometimes chronic care.

## Summary

We have seen how a therapist benefits from the social role as healer while using basic psychotherapeutic tactics. The healer role arises not only throughout the health care ecosystem but also within religion and popular culture. Although other features of this role are important— the safe environment, the theory or myth and the processes or ritual— the *therapeutic relationship* requires the most attention and care. So much depends on the therapeutic alliance that perhaps half of the desired behavioral improvement can be created by that element alone.

Basic psychotherapeutic tactics manifest themselves through successful communication using such simple devices as diction, naming and metacommunication. These techniques foster emotional experiences, improve cognitive understanding and consolidate beneficial changes in behavior that lead to a successful therapy outcome.

In the past, it was common to find a therapist wedded to a single psychotherapy. The chosen methodology was often supported by academic and political forces unrelated to the rate of successful outcomes. This one-size-fits-all approach has weakened in the face of the demonstrated success of so many "unorthodox" methodologies. Jane's approach to psychotherapy is best described as *eclectic*. She uses whatever therapy approach seems to best fit the clinical situation. Her decision as to what strategies are most promising depends on her ability to correctly formulate each case. When she is successful, as she was with Dorothy, Sally and Elizabeth, the therapy goes well. When her formulation is off the mark, problems arise, as they did with George and Charles. Her diverse approach, nevertheless, provides the best chance for positive outcomes with the widest variety of presented problems.

## References

Driessen, E., & Hollon, S. D. (2019). Cognitive-behavioral therapy for mood disorders: Efficacy, moderators and mediators. *Psychiatric Clinics of North America*, 33(3), 537–555.

HHS Press Office. (2022, January 25). *Treasury Issue 2022: Mental Health Parity and Addiction Equity Act Report to Congress*. US Departments of Labor, Health and Human Services.

# Glossary

**Acting out:** The behavioral expression of stressful thoughts, emotions or conflicts that the person feels unable or unwilling to put into words.

**Aim:** In a treatment plan, the desired overall best outcome the therapy seeks to achieve.

**Affective experiencing:** The elicitation of the emotional content of material brought out through the therapeutic process.

**Antecedents:** Events or historical influences that precede and have a causative relationship with current behaviors and symptoms. An important method of understanding current behavior, especially in cognitive-behavioral therapy.

**Auxiliary ego:** The therapist's supportive role in providing executive functions such as emotional support, intellectual processing and possibly advice to patients who lack these skills. The term is also used in psychodrama and other psychotherapies with different meanings.

**Behavioral regulation:** Significant and long-lasting positive behavioral change brought about by the therapeutic process.

**Borderline personality:** A disorder characterized by poor emotional control; problems with self-image; impulsivity; suicidal and self-destructive behavior; and fraught interpersonal relationships.

**Boundary violation:** A breach of the spoken or unspoken "rules" that govern the meeting between client and therapist. Example: a client who frequently attempts to overstay the end of the appointment.

**Catastrophize:**   To exaggerate the expected consequences of an internal thought or an external event, often to the extent of the worst possible outcome.

**Chronicle:**   A patient's recitation of unrelated and often inconsequential events leading up to the session, usually as a way of avoiding or resisting the work of therapy.

**Clarification:**   A step in the process of psychodynamic therapy that seeks to elaborate and make clear the meaning of a patient's behavior.

**Client-centered therapy:**   See "Rogers, Carl R."

**Clinical case management:**   A strategic intervention that provides a client with helpful suggestions about other sources of help.

**Cognitive-behavioral therapy (CBT):**   A therapeutic modality based on mechanisms of learning and information processing that focuses on the way environmental and internal conditions influence patient behavior.

**Cognitive mastery:**   The rational basis of a therapeutic modality that provides an intellectual framework for the therapeutic work.

**Confrontation:**   In psychodynamic therapy, the presentation to the patient of evidence underlying the cause or manifestation of a problematic behavior.

**Counterphobic:**   A defense mechanism in which the patient seeks out or plunges into anxiety-provoking situations in an effort to deny or overcome them. Example: a person with a fear of heights who goes bungee-jumping or sky-diving.

**Countertransference:**   The therapist's emotional response to a client based on the therapist's own history rather than a rational response based on the client's presentation.

**Diction:**   The choice of words and sentence construction that reflects the patient's intelligence and level of education in order to enhance effective communication and comprehension of the therapist's ideas.

**Directive:**   A group of therapies centered on prescribing exercises, behavior modifications, educational reading and the like in order to encourage changes in behavior.

**Dynamics:** The psychological forces behind the patient's ideation and behavior.

**Eclectic therapy:** An approach to psychotherapeutic treatment that tries to choose the most effective option among the wide variety of theories and techniques.

**Ego dystonic (ego alien):** Behaviors, values or emotions that conflict with the client's self-understanding or self-image.

**Ego syntonic:** Behaviors, values or emotions that are in harmony with the patient's self-understanding or self-image and are therefore more resistant to change.

**Existential crisis:** Emotional turmoil created by the client's recognition or apprehension of the idea that life may not have meaning, purpose or value, or that lack of personal freedom, loneliness, or death are unavoidable consequences of human existence.

**Formulation:** An explanation of the patient's problems, based on any psychological theory of behavioral disorders, used to provide a basis for construction of a treatment plan. As new information emerges in the course of treatment, the formulation must be revised, usually leading to greater accuracy and a more successful treatment plan.

**Foundation:** See "Lay a foundation."

**Goal:** In treatment planning, one of the objectives set in the plan to work toward the desired aim.

**Hypochondriasis:** An anxiety disorder characterized by the persistent idea that one has a serious or fatal illness without confirming medical evidence.

**Hypothesis:** A statement of probability about the antecedents or causes of a behavior that will be the focus of therapeutic intervention.

**Identification:** (1) The psychological attempt to model oneself after a portion of the behavior of another person, such as a child after a parent, a teenager after a celebrity or an employee after an admired supervisor. The imitated behavior may be a positive or negative aspect of the model; for example, an abused child may become a bully among peers. Sometimes called partial identification. (2)

The first step in psychodynamic therapy; namely, to call attention to a target symptom, habit or behavior.

**Intellectualization:**   A mechanism of defense in which apparently rational thinking is employed in the service of protecting a person from threatening emotional content.

**Interpretation:**   An explanation of behavior offered to a client about the source or cause of psychodynamic symptoms in order to initiate a helpful behavioral change.

**Introjected object:**   A form of identification in which the perceived qualities of another person (for example, a parent) are internalized and then treated as part of the self, sometimes with negative consequences.

**Isolation of affect:**   A mechanism of defense in which a patient blocks the emotion associated with a painful or traumatic event. Example: someone who relates the events of an assault without experiencing the fear, anger or grief associated with the attack.

**Lay a foundation:**   The process of preparation for an exploration of an important event or therapeutic intervention by eliciting its contextual or historical precursors.

**Metacommunication:**   A statement or question that responds to the type of communication rather than to its overt content. A response to the implication of a patient's statement rather than to its concrete message. Example: "What time is it?" "Are you in a hurry?"

**Microexpression:**   A brief involuntary facial expression that conveys the person's true emotional state of the moment. The observer may not consciously register the expression yet still pick up the affective state it conveys.

**Modeling:**   A covert feature of therapy that allows a client to incorporate certain positive perceived features of the therapist. See also: "Identification."

**Name, Rename, Reframe, Relabel:**   A therapeutic tactic that attempts to question or change the patient's attitude and perception of an event, an experience or another person by suggesting an alternative term with a different meaning or context.

**Negative overgeneralization (see also:** "Overgeneralization"): Reference to an exaggerated or overly broad judgment of the undesirable or dangerous effects of a life situation.

**Normative:**   The reference to a cultural, societal or group standard of expected behavior either to conform behavior or to judge behavior in others.

**Observing ego:**   Self-observation, the ability to monitor one's own thoughts, emotions, actions, defense and motivations, as well as what effect one's behavior has on another person. This ego function is usually a combination of both innate and learned function.

**Obsessional personality:**   The exaggeration of common traits, such as intellectualization, perfectionism, orderliness and control, that interfere with personal behavior and interpersonal relationships.

**Overgeneralization (see also:** "Negative overgeneralization"): A cognitive distortion that needlessly or falsely applies a single instance to many or all similar situations. The application of a conclusion about anything that applies it to more situations than are called for. Sometimes called black or white thinking.

**Overvalued idea:**   A false belief that is maintained despite strong evidence that it is untrue.

**Paradoxical intention or intervention:**   The deliberate use of conflicting instructions that have the effect of reversing a symptom, habit or other behavior.

**Passive-aggressive:**   The indirect expression of negative feelings, such as anger, resentment and frustration, often as a way of controlling others or to avoid the consequences of a personal or social response. Example: someone who procrastinates in order to defy the controlling behavior of an authority without challenging it directly.

**Placebo effect:**   A beneficial effect from an inert or non-therapeutic source. Example: a patient whose presenting symptom improves when placed on the waiting list for treatment.

**Provoked emotion:**   The therapist's emotional response to a client's attempt to elicit it in order to justify the client's problems or to manipulate the therapist in a way favorable to the client's needs. Example: a therapist who feels angry at the stubborn silence of a client who is testing to see if the therapist "really cares."

**Psychodynamic:**   In psychotherapy, the hypothesis that current behaviors are influenced or caused by past emotional experience.

**Rename, Reframe, Relabel:**   See "Name."

**Real relationship:**   Those aspects of the interaction between therapist and patient that are based on their conventional status and involving the administrative, non-therapeutic aspects of their association. Example: the financial arrangement in which the patient pays the therapist for services rendered.

**Regression:**   A maladaptive response to stress or conflict that provokes earlier, more primitive and less effective responses to perceived danger.

**Resistance:**   The client's obstruction or avoidance of therapeutic interventions, especially those that require a change in behavior.

**Rhetoric:**   An important component of effective communication that utilizes examples, stories, metaphors and other devices to convey the importance of a therapeutic idea.

**Rogers, Carl R. (1902–1987):**   An American psychologist who developed "client-centered" therapy, an approach designed to help patient's "self-actualize" that requires the therapist to be real and authentic (congruence), to be non-judgmental (unconditional positive regard) and to show empathy by reflecting the client's experience (accurate empathic understanding).

**Secondary gain:**   The reinforcement of problematic behavior or particular symptoms by the advantages perceived by the patient, usually unconsciously, from remaining in the "sick role."

**Sociopathic personality:**   Also termed antisocial personality. A person who lacks empathy and uses intelligence, lying and charm to manipulate others for personal gain. The sociopathic person may use threats and aggression to control others. Relationships are superficial and one-sided: the other person is often treated like an object for personal gratification without consideration or reciprocity.

**Strategy:**   A therapeutic system employed to achieve a specific goal. Example: cognitive-behavioral therapy.

**Structural impasse:**   A loss of progress in a therapeutic endeavor brought about by failures in the therapeutic alliance or the treatment contract. If not overcome, an impasse will result in treatment failure.

**Symptomatic act:**   A behavior that conveys an otherwise unexpressed implication or message that the client does not consciously wish to reveal. For example, a young man who constantly trips himself on the rug coming into the office may express the idea, "I'm stumbling through life."

**Tactic:**   In treatment planning, the specific intervention chosen, usually among others, to achieve a goal of the plan. Example: in psychodynamic psychotherapy the presentation of an interpretation.

**Therapeutic alliance:**   The positive, cooperative and collaborative relationship engendered by the therapist's overt desire to help the client and the client's perception of the therapist's expertise that engenders a willingness to seek change in the client's problematic behaviors.

**Therapeutic contract:**   The agreement between therapist and patient of what the therapy will try to achieve and what steps may be needed to reach it. An overt enumeration of these steps provides a firm foundation on which the contemplated therapy can proceed.

**Transactional:**   An interpersonal relationship based on both parties' anticipated receipt of benefits.

**Transference:**   The distortion of the client's attitude toward and relationship with the therapist that occurs when experiences, feelings and expectations from an earlier relationship are projected onto the therapist. Example: the belief that the therapist is punitive and judgmental based on the client's experience during childhood of a parent with those characteristics.

**Treatment plan:**   The construction of a template of expected outcome from therapy that includes identification of goals, choice of a strategy for achieving each of them and consideration of tactics needed to carry them out. The initial plan may need revision as additional history emerges through the therapeutic process. (See also: "Formulation.")

**Why questions:**   A problematic phrasing of a request for information by the therapist because of its implication of criticism, disapproval or even condemnation that may unintentionally damage the therapeutic alliance.

**Working through:**   The therapeutic process of repetition that promotes behavioral change.

**Working alliance:**   See "Therapeutic alliance."

# Index